Rosemary Gladstar's
MEDICINAL
HERBS A Beginner's Guide

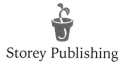

Storey Publishing

The mission of Storey Publishing is to serve our customers by
publishing practical information that encourages
personal independence in harmony with the environment.

Edited by Deborah Balmuth and Nancy Ringer
Art direction and book design by Jessica Armstrong

Cover photography © Jason Houston: front (top left & right, bottom left), back
(all); © koi88/Dreamstime.com: front (bottom center); © Saxon Holt: front
(top center, bottom right)
Interior photography by © Jason Houston, except as noted on page 218

Indexed by Nancy D. Wood

Storey Publishing
210 MASS MoCA Way
North Adams, MA 01247
www.storey.com

Printed in the United States by Versa Press
20 19 18 17

LIBRARY OF CONGRESS CATALOGING-IN-PUBLICATION DATA

Gladstar, Rosemary.
  Rosemary Gladstar's medicinal herbs : a beginner's guide / by Rosemary Gladstar.
    p. cm.
  Includes index.
  ISBN 978-1-61212-005-8 (pbk. : alk. paper)
  1. Herbs—Therapeutic use. 2. Materia medica, Vegetable.
  I. Title. II. Title: Medicinal herbs.
  RM666.H33G538 2012
  615.3'21—dc23
                    2011053101

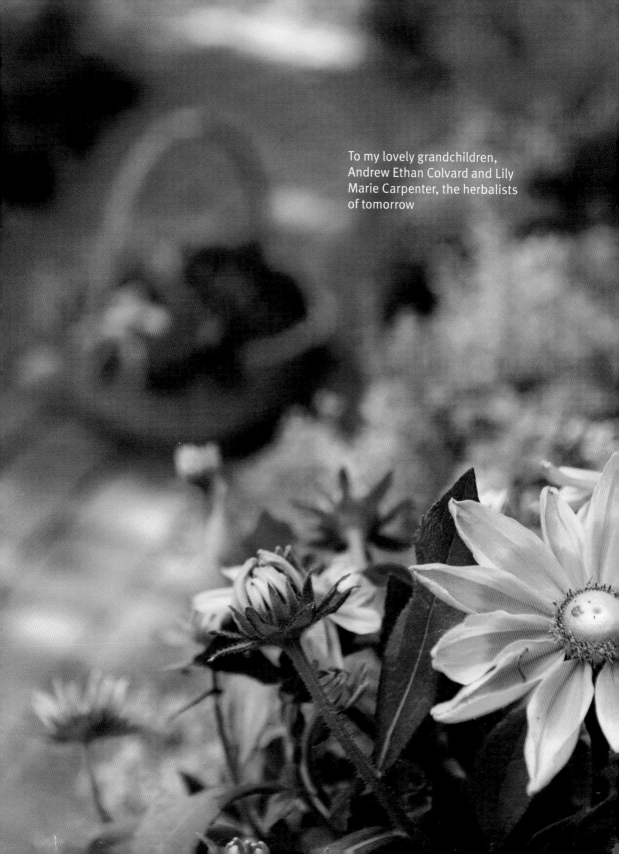

To my lovely grandchildren, Andrew Ethan Colvard and Lily Marie Carpenter, the herbalists of tomorrow

CONTENTS

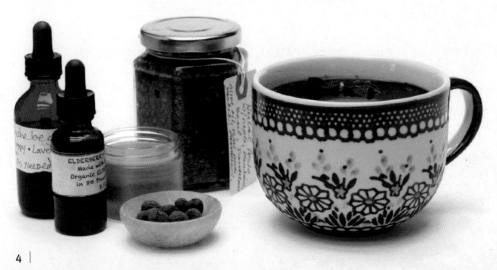

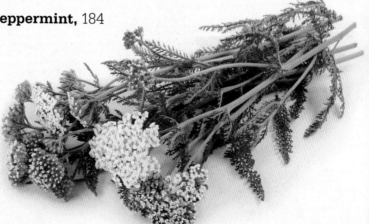

CHAPTER 1

Welcome to the Wonderful World of Medicinal Herbs

RECOGNIZED AS THE OLDEST SYSTEM OF HEALING on the planet, herbal medicine traces its roots back to the earliest civilizations. Today, herbalism continues to flourish as a people's healing art. Even with the amazing technological advances of conventional (allopathic) medicine, herbalism — the art and science of healing with plants — is still widely popular. And its popularity is gaining, not waning. According to the World Health Organization, 80 percent of the world's population used some form of traditional medicine in 2008, and its rate of affordability, availability, and accessibility is surging.

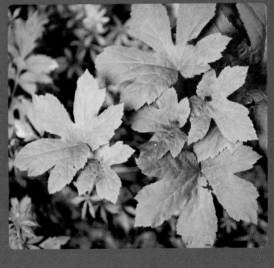

So it's no wonder you're drawn to these healing plants and curious to learn more about them. But perhaps you're nervous about trying herbal home remedies: What are these herbs? Are they safe? Do they work? Can you grow them at home? Can you make your own remedies? When and how do you use them? How easy is it to get started? These are some of questions we'll address in this book.

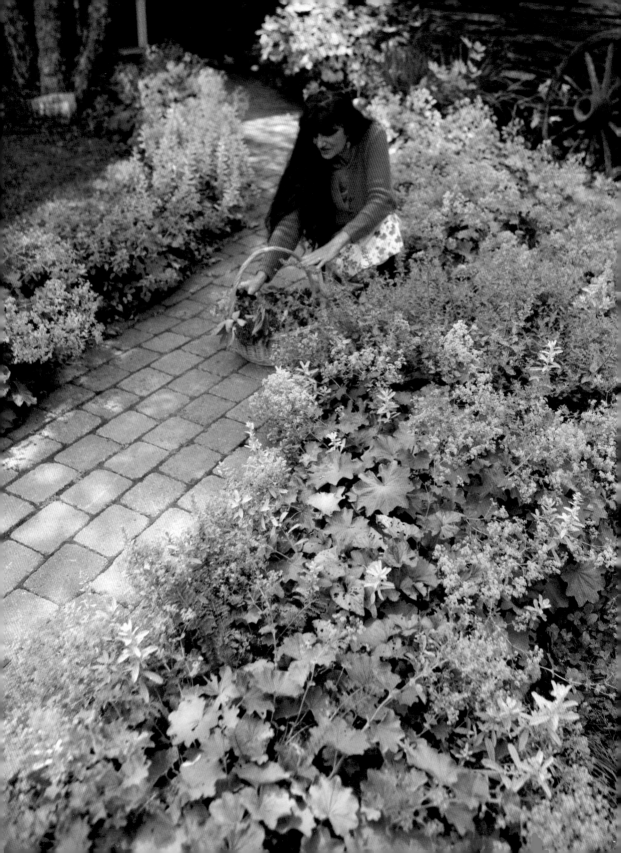

My Story

I was one of the lucky ones. When I was a child, my grandmother took me into the fields and showed me the wild plants she knew. Quietly, with a gentle but stern voice, she taught me their healing powers. When she weeded her garden, I was often kneeling beside her, watching her carefully sort the plants she pulled. I learned early which herbs went into the edibles basket and which went into the compost, and, as importantly, I learned why.

We were a farm family growing up in the wake of World War II. Resilient, hardy, and handy, we were taught to use what was available, useful, and inexpensive. Herbal remedies were one of those things. My grandmother had up her sleeve an armory of useful herbal remedies that she had learned over a long and difficult lifetime. She was a survivor of the Armenian genocide of World War I, and she told us grandkids that it had been her knowledge of plants and her faith in God that saved her life.

As kids, we suffered few illnesses or accidents that our grandmother and parents weren't able to treat effectively at home with herbal remedies. In fact, I recall only two incidents that required a doctor's care: when my younger sister swallowed rat poison (she survived, by the way) and when my older sister fell off the family horse and broke her hip. Not a bad record for a family with

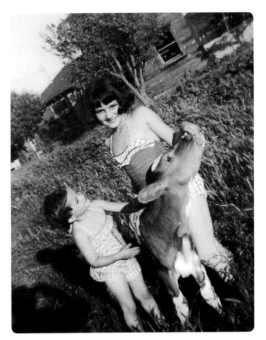

Here I am with my younger sister and one of the calves on our family farm.

BOTANICAL BOOM

According to *The Natural Pharmacy*, by Schuyler Lininger et al., one out of every three adult Americans uses complementary/alternative medical care. Sales of botanicals have increased more than 300 percent since the 1990s and currently are an $8 billion industry.

five active farm children . . . and good testament to the effectiveness of herbal home remedies.

What Is a Medicinal Herb?

If you use herbs in cooking, then you've already taken the first step in using herbal medicine. All of our common culinary herbs and spices are among our most important and esteemed herbal medicines. And if you garden, tucking herbs here and there in your vegetable and flower beds for their added scent and beauty, then you also have been "practicing" herbal medicine.

Garden herbs such as lavender, thyme, sage, basil, rosemary, mint, yarrow, and peppermint are some of our most trusted herbal medicines and have long histories of use as teas, salves, poultices, and tinctures for healing purposes. Open your refrigerator and you may find more common herbal remedies, including horseradish (one of the best remedies for sinus infections) and cabbage (a singularly effective poultice for shingles and hives).

But wait, you might say, aren't some of these plants vegetables and not herbs? Botanically speaking, an herb is an herbaceous plant with a nonwoody stem. However, when herbalists speak of medicinal herbs, they are basically including any plant that can be used in healing. Remember, herbalism is an art that evolved over centuries around people and people's needs. It only makes sense that people would use what they had available, in the kitchen or in the backyard. Many of the most common plants are still our best and most popular remedies for common ailments.

So even without knowing it, you may already be a practitioner of herbal home medicine.

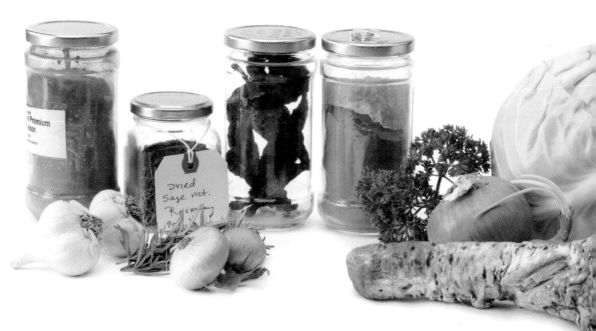

How Is Herbal Medicine Used?

While conventional or allopathic medicine is particularly effective in life-threatening situations and unrivaled in its ability to save lives, herbal medicine is the medicine of the home. It is used most effectively for the myriad non-emergency health problems that arise in everyday life: simple first-aid situations, the bumps and bruises of life, headaches, colds and fevers and flu, coughs and aches and pains, and chronic illness.

But more important than "curing" illnesses, plants play a great role in preventing them. Rich in nutrients, herbs are the supreme preventive medicine, bolstering our body's ability to fight off pathogens that cause illness. How do they do this?

In addition to having superconcentrations of the important nutrients essential to the health of the human body, medicinal plants tend to be concentrated in specific chemicals that aid and abet the human immune system. When we eat medicinal plants, our own body becomes more resilient, hardy, and persistent, like the tenacious weedy plant that seems able to survive anything, from endless mowing to barrages of nasty "weed killers."

BALANCING ALLOPATHIC & HERBAL MEDICINE

Make no mistake, this book is about family herbalism. It is written as an introduction to using herbs to enhance health and well-being and to reintroduce the traditional practice of home health care for everyday common illnesses. But it does not advocate that herbs or home remedies be used to replace the guidance of trained health-care professionals.

Health problems that are beyond the care of a home herbalist include life-threatening illnesses such as heart disease and kidney disease, neurological disorders, clinical depression and anxiety, broken bones, poisoning, and life-threatening injuries such as gunshot wounds, wounds with excessive bleeding, and so on. Any life-threatening injury or illness should always be treated under the supervision of a competent medical professional.

A good rule of thumb to follow is that any injury or illness that does not respond to herbal remedies and home health care in a timely manner should be evaluated by a professional health-care practitioner. If an injury or illness gets worse, not better, then seek professional help. If you don't feel comfortable using herbal remedies to treat a particular injury or illness, then seek help.

One of the major differences between conventional (allopathic) medicine and herbal or natural medicine lies in their relationship to constitutional or foundational wellness. Conventional medicine, as we all know, is great for treating acute illness and can often temporarily alleviate its symptoms. Such treatment can be extremely comforting to someone in the midst of an "attack": an asthma attack, for instance, or an oncoming migraine. However, symptom suppression, while necessary, hardly means the cause or root of the illness has been addressed.

Herbs and natural therapies are the medicine of choice for fostering constitutional wellness and addressing the root of chronic health problems. Chronic issues — meaning they are long term and/or recurring — usually have their root in lifestyle choices, environmental conditions, and/or genetics. They are most often corrected by lifestyle changes that include dietary changes, herbal remedies, and exercise programs. Treat the root or core of the problem, and the whole gets healthier.

Thankfully, we don't have to make the choice between conventional medicine and herbal medicine. Both are amazing, effective systems of healing, yet they are distinctly different systems, designed to be used in different situations. Each is complementary to the other.

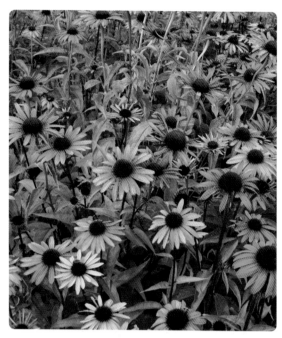

A field of echinacea can provide a wealth of immune-boosting remedies.

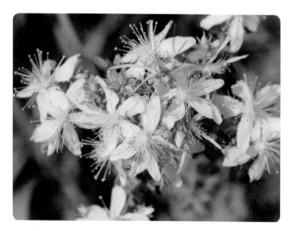

The flowers of St. John's wort have medicinal properties that are useful for relieving stress and anxiety.

The Benefits of Herbal Medicine

One of the greatest benefits of herbal medicine is that it gives us the ability to become more self-reliant. Feeling that we have choices in how we care for ourselves and our families, and that we ourselves can play a central role in treatment and preventive medicine, can help us build a positive attitude of empowerment. With very little effort, time, or money, we can grow our own herbs, make our own medicines, and care for our families and ourselves, much as people have been doing for millennia. Herbalism is truly an accessible, inexpensive, natural, gentle, and, most importantly, effective system of healing.

Herbs are among the safest medicines available. This does not mean that there are no herbs with harmful side effects. There are, but they are an isolated group, and most of them are unavailable commercially. Occasionally an herb will stimulate an idiosyncratic, or individual, reaction in a person. This doesn't mean the herb is toxic; it's just a poor choice for that particular individual. Strawberries, a perfectly delicious fruit, are a sweet treat for some and a noxious poison for others.

Herbs are also an inexpensive way to boost your health. Herbal supplements for sale in a natural foods store are, capsule by capsule, much less expensive than pharmaceuticals. And herbal medicine becomes really cost effective and inexpensive when you plant some herbs, don an apron, and brew up your own remedies. You'll be surprised to discover how easy, inexpensive, and fun it is to make your own salves, tinctures, syrups, capsules, and teas, especially if you're making them from herbs you've grown yourself! Begin by making simple medicines for coughs, colds, cuts, infections, and sprains, and you'll find they not only work wonderfully but can also cut the cost of family health care, in the same way that growing your own vegetables helps reduce your grocery bills.

A MANTRA FOR HOME HEALTH CARE

I am my own healer. I have a radiant voice within that guides me. I can make decisions for myself. I can rely on others as needed, but at my discretion. It is my body, my health, my balance, and my responsibility to make right choices for myself. Right choices include working with competent health-care professionals when necessary, allowing friends and family to help as needed, and, above all, being true to my beliefs, with the wisdom and willingness to change as part of the path of healing.

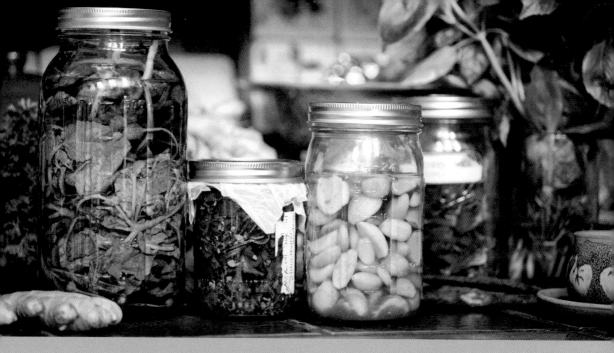

SIDE EFFECTS?

I once heard a doctor state that the "side effects" of pharmaceutical medication are not side effects at all, but the actual effects of the medication. This is an aspect I appreciate about herbal remedies; they are effective, yes, but side effects are few and far between. There are people who have idiosyncratic reactions to certain foods and herbs, but it's an individual reaction rather than toxicity in the plants. And while there certainly are toxic plants that can have nasty "side effects" or actions, most of these herbs are not legal for use and certainly are not used in herbal family medicine. In this book you'll find none of the herbs with a potential for toxicity, but rather those congenial herbs with a long history of use as food and medicine with few or no known side effects.

When a person does experience "side effects" from a particular herb, they are generally short term and idiosyncratic: itchy eyes, sore throat, a skin rash, or nausea and an upset stomach. These symptoms disappear after discontinuance of the offending herb and are not long lasting.

Because we are working with nontoxic herbs with few or no side effects, we don't have to be as careful with exact dosages. The problem is generally not taking enough of the herbs to be effective, rather than taking too much.

Starting a Home Medicine Garden

Whether you're growing vegetables, herbs, or flowers, one of the greatest joys of gardening is the connection you make with nature. As you tend your garden, you observe the rhythms and cycles of nature, watching a tiny seed grow to maturity, flower, and, perhaps, seed again. This understanding of natural rhythms and cycles is integral to most traditional systems of healing. Perhaps it's one of the big disconnects we feel with modern medicine: we have little connection to where drugs come from, how they are made, and who makes them. By starting a little herb garden, you set up a direct connection with the earth and the healing plants it nurtures. You are also assured of quality herbs that are grown "nature's way."

If you've never attempted growing herbs, not to worry. It's really quite easy. Most medicinal plants are "weedy" in nature; they define hardiness and have a knack for growing even in adverse conditions. Given the right soil, light, and water, herbs generally thrive.

As recently as a 100 years ago, almost every American household had a kitchen garden with an "apothecary" section designated for healing plants. It's fun to re-create these traditional gardens. Dig up a small plot by the back door, plant your favorite medicinal herbs (and edible herbs as well), and step back in time.

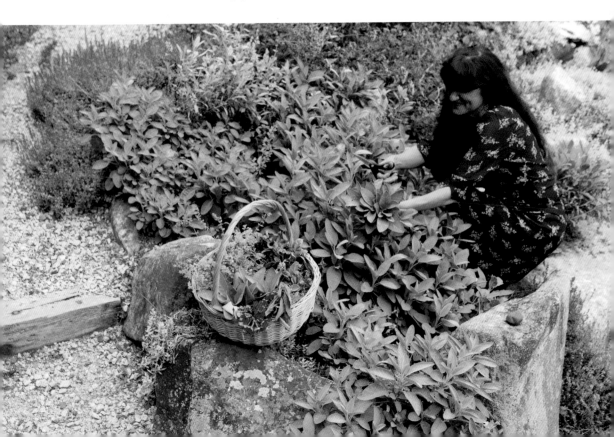

Medicinal herbs can also easily be woven into the tapestry of an already-established garden. For instance, echinacea, yarrow, and valerian are lovely additions to flower gardens, providing color, scent, and beauty. Calendula, chamomile, and thyme are often planted in vegetable gardens as "companion" plants, said to enhance the growth and vitality of their vegetable partners. Still other medicinal herbs, such as basil, parsley, and dill, are common culinary herbs, often found in their own patch known as the herb garden. And, of course, there's the lawn that surrounds most homes. Reclaiming a section of lawn for a small plot of medicinal herbs is a revolutionary act that may get your neighbors talking.

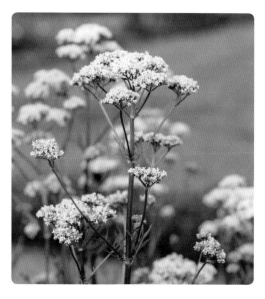

It's surprising to discover that some of our most highly prized herbal medicine is found in familiar flowering herbs such as valerian.

Soil Health

Soil health is the key to good gardening. Good soil is like gold to the gardener. If you see a lot of earthworms in your soil, then it's probably healthy. If not, you may need to do some "soil doctoring" before you plant your garden.

Herbs don't require an overly rich soil or lots of fertilizer or soil amendments; they are not big eaters. But the idea that they will be more potent if grown in nutrient-poor soil and made to struggle is a myth. Medicinal plants, like any other plants, need good, healthy soil in order to develop fully.

To build healthy soil, amend it with organic compost and well-aged manure. If it tends to be clumpy and thick, rather than rich and friable, add sand as well. If you see a healthy garden in your neighborhood, ask your neighbors what they've done to their soil. Or ask for recommendations at a local nursery. But be sure that whatever you add to your soil is organic. Nonorganic soil and soil amendments might grow plants that look healthy, but ultimately chemical additives are no better for the soil and the ecosystem than they are for our health.

As Tammi Hartung writes in her book *Homegrown Herbs,* "Plants utilize nutrients in the soil to become vibrant and healthy, and producing vital soil is the first important step toward a gorgeous and useful herb garden." Tammi's book contains a wonderful chapter devoted to building great soil, and it's well worth reading.

Garden Designs

Keep designs simple. If you've never gardened before, try a ladder or wagon-wheel design. Lay an old wooden ladder or wagon wheel over well-prepared soil (cleared, forked, amended, and otherwise worked as needed). Add more soil to fill in the spaces between the ladder rungs or wheel spokes, and work the soil in. Plant a single type of herb in each rung. This simple and popular design is lovely, makes weeding easy, and allows the plants to grow fully. It's a fun project for kids as well.

Raised beds are very popular now, especially in urban areas, where soil health may be questionable due to years of lawn fertilizers, chemical residues, and other types of pollution. Most nurseries and many home garden centers sell ready-made raised beds that are simple to assemble. There's no excuse for not being handy here — even I can assemble these beds! And it's amazing how many medicinal plants can be grown in some of the space-saving designs that are available. Try the circular raised beds with multiple tiers. They are lovely filled with medicinal herbs, flowers, and vegetables and enable you to plant an amazingly large garden in a very small space. If you are a true handyperson, then you can build a raised bed with nothing more than 2×6s and a few nails. Or you can use bricks, cinder blocks, or even just dirt that's raised and formed into mounds.

The idea is to start simple: good dirt, a few plants, and you're ready to go. Experience success and become garden impassioned!

Some medicinal herbs that are easy to grow and will do well in a simple ladder or wagon-wheel design and/or in raised beds are:

» Basil
» Calendula
» Cayenne
» Chamomile
» Chickweed
» Dandelion
» Echinacea
» Garlic
» Lavender
» Lemon balm
» Licorice
» Oats
» Peppermint
» Plantain
» Red clover
» Rosemary
» Sage
» St. John's wort
» Spearmint
» Thyme
» Yarrow

The following herbs are easy to grow as well, but they get very large and may quickly overtake a small garden design. You might want to plant them at the edge of the garden:

» Burdock
» Marsh mallow
» Mullein
» Valerian

CONTAINER GARDENS

If you don't have space for a garden, many medicinal herbs do quite well in containers. Placed on a sunny patio, along a driveway, or in a sunny window, they can add fragrance and beauty as well as provide inexpensive medicine. These potted plants can be moved about to get better sunlight as the seasons change and can be moved indoors for winter storage. Some of these herbs will happily grow year-round indoors.

Not all herbs, however, like to be confined to a pot, so check with your local nursery and see which herbs are most likely to do well in the confinement of a container.

In general, some medicinal plants that can be grown easily in containers are:

- Basil
- Calendula
- Cayenne
- Chamomile
- Chickweed
- Dandelion
- Echinacea
- Garlic
- Ginger
- Lavender
- Lemon balm
- Peppermint
- Plantain
- Red clover
- Rosemary
- Sage
- St. John's wort
- Spearmint
- Thyme
- Turmeric
- Yarrow

Know Your Local Weeds

For *really* inexpensive herbal medicine, learn your local weeds! Free for the picking, many common "weeds" are excellent medicinal herbs. The earliest European settlers of the North American continent brought with them burdock, dandelion, nettle, plantain, and valerian, which they relied on for food and medicine. Most of these plants settled nicely into the local landscape (or in some cases took it over), and they are among our most popular herbal remedies today.

There are also many native North American plants that were used by the indigenous peoples in sophisticated systems of healing. But many of these native medicinals, like the people who used them, are at risk and/or endangered. Before harvesting any native medicinal plants from the wild, check with local native-plant societies and your state's department of natural resources. Many offer lists of regional endangered plants online. Consider becoming involved in the work of United Plant Savers, a group dedicated to the conservation and cultivation of native medicinal herbs (see Resources).

There are many excellent books on wild plant identification, but the very best way to learn your "wild neighbors" is to go on a plant-identification walk with a local expert. An afternoon spent "herb walking" is always an enjoyable experience, and one that is often addictive!

Harvesting Medicinal Herbs

The different parts of plants should be harvested at different times. Follow these general guidelines.

BUDS AND FLOWERS are best harvested just as they are opening. Don't wait for them to open fully; by that point, they will have lost much of their medicinal potency. For instance, St. John's wort buds are perfect when they are fully formed but not fully opened.

LEAVES usually are best harvested before a plant is in full bloom. This is only a very general guideline, though; for some plants, like many of the mints, the leaves are often more potent when the plants are in flower. How can you tell? Examine the leaves. Are they in their prime? Do they taste strong? Are they colorful? Is there little insect damage? Use the same discretion you would apply to selecting greens from the produce department. Do they seem alive, vital, and healthy? Then harvest!

ROOTS are best dug in the fall or spring, when the energy of the plant is still stored in the root or bulb. As spring and summer unfold, the plant's energy moves upward to provide nourishment for the leaves, flowers, and seed or fruit, leaving the root less potent.

These are just general guidelines and, as such, are to be taken with a grain of salt. Always assess the quality of each herb you'll be harvesting, and select the best time for each plant based on when it's in its prime. Much like when you're shopping for produce, you just *know* when the fruit has been picked too early or has been stored too long. Develop this same instinct with medicinal plants. Use your senses to determine quality.

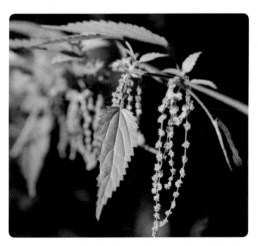

Harvest nettle leaf early in the season before the plant begins to flower or go to seed.

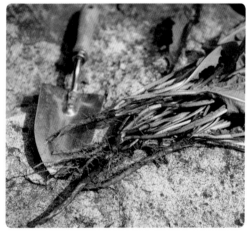

Dandelion roots are best harvested in the spring or fall, but they can be usefully dug up anytime during the growing season.

Drying High-Quality Herbs

Once you've harvested your medicinal herbs, you may want to dry some to preserve them for future use. The best drying conditions for herbs are:

» A steady warm temperature of around 90° to 110°F

» Minimal humidity: the less, the better

» Good airflow

» Protection from direct sunlight

Keep these points in mind and you'll have good-quality dried herbs for year-round use.

Though it's easy to dry herbs, there are some challenges. Heat and humidity are important factors. Many of the medicinal constituents in plants are heat sensitive, especially the aromatic essential oils. Drying plants in temperatures above 110°F can cause these compounds to dissipate. And if you're trying to air-dry herbs in high humidity or during a "rainy season," good luck! You'll have better luck using a food dryer or dehydrator.

The traditional method for drying herbs is to hang them in small bundles from rafters. Though this is a quaint and lovely way to display them, it's not

FRESH VS. DRIED

There is nothing quite as good as the taste of fresh-picked herbs. But high-quality dried herbs can be as effective as fresh herbs in teas and other herbal products. The emphasis here is on *high quality*. If herbs are picked at their prime, dried quickly and at the right temperature, then packaged and stored correctly, the integrity of the fresh plants is preserved. All that's lost is the water content.

While herbalists generally emphasize using fresh herbs when they're available, there are times when dried herbs are preferable; for instance, when you're making salves and oils, it's better to use dried herbs because the water content in fresh plants can spoil the oil. Dried plants are often more concentrated than fresh

herbs, again because the diluting water content has been removed, and this can be an advantage in medicine making. But probably the best reason to use dried herbs is that fresh herbs are not available year-round and, for most of us, some of our favorite medicinal plants are not grown locally.

The rule of thumb is to use fresh herbs when possible, but high-quality dried herbs will do just fine (and in some cases are favored). One thing that's not arguable is that you should use organically grown herbs whenever possible, even though the cost may be a bit more. After all, you are using your herbal remedies for health and healing; it's best not to have them laced with pesticides and herbicides.

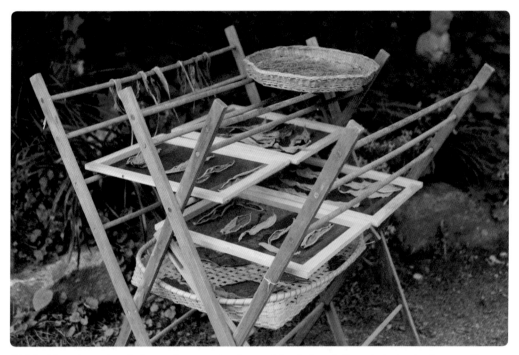

Old-fashioned wooden drying racks are not only great for drying clothes, but also herbs as well. Place the drying rack in a shaded, warm area of either the house or yard and layer baskets or screens filled with herbs on the shelves.

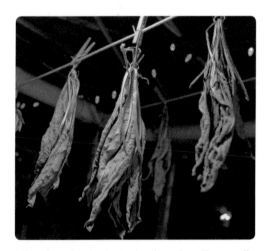

When hanging herbs to dry, keep bundles small and well-spaced so herbs dry evenly and quickly. Be sure to take them down as soon as they are completely dry so they don't gather dust and insects.

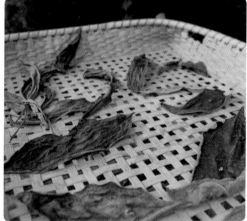

When drying herbs in baskets or on screens, place herbs in single layers so they get plenty of air circulation and warmth. If layered on top of one another, they often turn moldy from lack of circulation.

always the most efficient way to dry them. The herbs tend to be left hanging too long, far past their drying time; either they're forgotten or they become a touch of old-fashioned decor, and they overdry and gather dust. If you do decide to dry herbs in bundles, keep the bundles small so the herbs dry thoroughly and quickly, and take the bundles down as soon as they are completely dry.

Though there are a few challenges to drying high-quality herbs, it's a skill that anyone can master.

Baskets and screens are great for drying herbs. Select ones that allow for good airflow. In a warm, dry spot in your house, set them across two chairs, stools, sawhorses, or whatever else you have on hand to hold them up, or tie ribbons or strings to them and hang them. If the spot gets a lot of sunlight, cover the drying area with a light porous cloth. Popular among herbalists are lightly woven nesting baskets that are specially made for drying herbs. They can be suspended one above the other, creating several tiers of baskets that allow for lots of drying space in a small area.

And, of course, you can dry herbs in a food dehydrator. But remember to set the temperature low (90° to 110°F).

No matter which method you use, once the herbs are dry, store them in glass jars with tight-fitting lids in a cool area protected from direct light. If stored properly, dried herbs will retain their medicinal qualities for at least a year, and sometimes much longer. You can tell whether an herb is still viable by its color, scent, and effectiveness; it should look, smell, and work just as it did on the day it finished drying.

Freezing Herbs

Freezing is another great way to preserve medicinal herbs, and it's the simplest method. Most herbs retain their medicinal properties, color, and taste when frozen. Some may lose their color or texture, but most are still flavorful and medicinal. Basil, for instance, is extremely sensitive to the cold. When frozen, its color changes to a deep dark purple or green, and it becomes mushy when defrosted. But it does retain most of its flavor and can be used in medicinal soups, teas, and other preparations in which its texture and color will not be noticed.

You can freeze herbs chopped or whole in ziplock bags. Or you may want to purée them (with a little water, if needed) and freeze the purée in ice-cube trays. When the purée is frozen, pop out the cubes and store them in ziplock bags. You can even purée together mixtures of fresh medicinal herbs for ready-made tea blends. Just drop one frozen cube into a cup of hot water and voilà! Instant, "almost fresh" tea.

How to Make Your Own Herbal Remedies

JOIN ME IN THE KITCHEN! If you know how to cook, you can make effective herbal remedies. Even if you're a novice in the kitchen, you can still make great herbal remedies. Though there is an art and science to making herbal medicine that can only be perfected over time, it's easy enough that often your first remedies will be nearly as good as those you make 20 years from now. As your knowledge and understanding of the plants expand, your ability to work with them also deepens. Relationship has as much to do with healing as exact

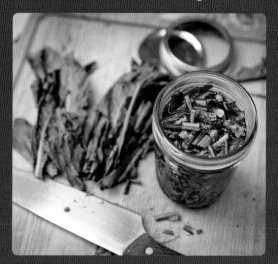

measurements, ingredients, and temperature. Making home herbal remedies is simple, fun, and easy, and the quality of the products you can make yourself in your own wondrous kitchen is as good as that of any product you can purchase, once you learn a few basic steps.

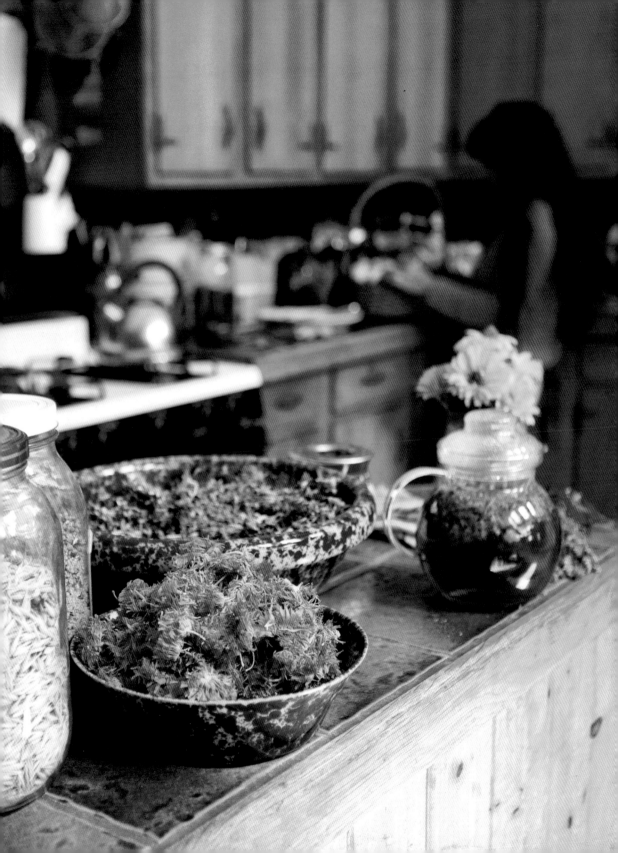

Setting Up Your Kitchen Pharmacy

In this chapter, I'll describe how to make six basic medicinal herbal preparations: teas, syrups, oils, salves, tinctures, and pills. Master these and you'll be able to address most, if not all, everyday health concerns. If you become inspired in the art of herbal preparation, as many are, you can continue the craft of herbal pharmacy and learn to make variations on the preparations presented here. Many small and large herbal companies began just this way, with a favorite herbal remedy brewed up in someone's kitchen.

Equipment & Supplies

What do we need to get started? Not much. A kitchen with basic tools will supply you with most of what you need to prepare herbal products. Some items I've found especially useful are:

>> Cheesecloth or muslin for straining out herbs
>> A large stainless-steel, double-meshed strainer
>> Stainless-steel pots with tight-fitting lids, including a double boiler
>> A grater reserved for grating beeswax
>> A variety of glass jars with lids for storing herbs, tinctures, salves, and so on
>> Measuring cups (though, honestly, I hardly ever use them)
>> A coffee grinder reserved for grinding herbs (Don't use your herb grinder for coffee; you'll forever have the scent of coffee in your herbs.)

NOTE: *Though I recommend stainless steel, other good materials for cooking pots include glass, ceramic, cast iron, and enamel. You'll hear arguments for and against any of these, depending on whom you talk to. But rather than get fanatical, do as Carl Jung, the famous psychologist, did: talk to your pots and select those that say "good morning" back. One of the few rules that most herbalists agree on is never to use aluminum pots and pans for preparing herbs, as heat releases microscopic amounts of toxic substances from the aluminum.*

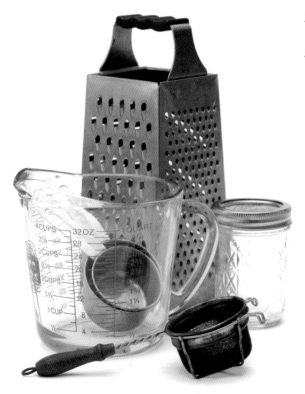

A SIMPLER MEASURE

While many people have converted to the metric system, I've reverted to the simpler's method of measuring. The term *simpler* is an old one, used in times past to refer to herbalists who worked with with only one or two plants at a time. Many modern herbalists use the simpler's system because it is both sensible and versatile. The simpler's measurement is a "part": for example, 3 parts chamomile, 2 parts oats, 1 part lemon balm. The formula defines the relationship among the ingredients, not exact amounts. The "part" is whatever unit of measure you desire; you simply have to apply it consistently. For instance, if you decide in this case to define *part* as an ounce, you would use 3 ounces of chamomile, 2 ounces of oats, and 1 ounce of

lemon balm. This would give you 6 ounces of an herbal tea blend. If you wanted to make a smaller amount, you could use a tablespoon as your definition of *part*: 3 tablespoons of chamomile, 2 tablespoons of oats, and 1 tablespoon of lemon balm. (Whatever the "part," it's best to use either all fresh herbs or all dried herbs, to maintain the ratio of active constituents.)

Although the simpler's method is not always perfectly exact, it is exacting enough to make excellent herbal products. And remember, because you're not using any ingredients with the potential for toxicity, you don't need to be as exact with your measurements. I often use the "pinch of this and dab of that" method of measuring with great success.

Sample formulas blended in the simpler's method

PARTS	PARTS IN TABLESPOONS	PARTS IN TEASPOONS
3 parts chamomile	3 tablespoons chamomile	3 teaspoons chamomile
2 parts oats	2 tablespoons oats	2 teaspoon oats
1 part lemon balm	1 tablespoon lemon balm	1 teaspoon lemon balm

Best Practices for Success

How do you make good herbal medicine? Some of the secrets to success are the similar to those any good cook would use in the kitchen.

LABEL YOUR PRODUCT IMMEDIATELY. Include on each label the following:

» The name of the product

» The date made

» A list of all ingredients, starting with the principal ingredients and finishing with the least significant

» Instructions for use, including whether the remedy is meant to be used internally or externally

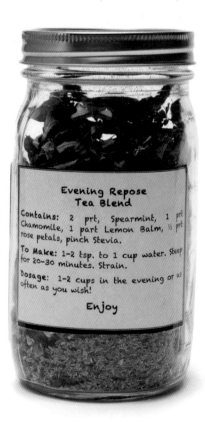

Today, with electronic labeling programs, you can design a professional-looking label yourself. Personalized labels are attractive and fun, and they add a nice touch to the finished product. Or, if you're not into playing Martha, you can make quick, easy, and inexpensive labels with colorful masking tape and a permanent marker.

KEEP GOOD RECORDS. Unfortunately, I've not always followed my own wise advice in this matter. I've created many an excellent product that could be savored only once because I could not remember that one special ingredient that went into it. Even today, in my well-stocked herbal pantry, I sometimes find myself staring in bewilderment at an unlabeled bottle that I recall quite clearly setting there months ago, thinking there was no way I would forget what I put in it. Such a waste, because you certainly can't use a product if you don't know what it is or what's in it. You will be far more satisfied if you organize your preparations as suggested, rather than following the example of this disorganized herbalist.

So keep a recipe file of all your products in your favorite format, whether on cards, in a medicine-making journal, or in a database. Record not only the ingredients but also the mode of preparation, including the dates of when you started making it, strained it, finished it, and so on, along with any notes that might be important: for example, the type of oil you used, whether you solar-infused it or cooked it on the stove, the ratio of herb to liquid. If you happen to make a remarkable herbal remedy that your friends rave about, it would be nice if you could re-create it, and that's what your notebook will help you do. It's especially delightful for grandchildren and younger generations to discover. That's not why we keep records, of course, but there's a sweet bit of satis-faction in knowing that this is how most of our information about herbalism has been passed down for generations, and now you're part of that thread.

TEST SMALL BATCHES. When making any remedy for the first time, make it in a small batch. It is better to lose only a few ingredients than an entire batch if your experimentation goes awry.

CHOOSE QUALITY HERBS. Ideally, you'd grow the herbs you're going to use in your own garden. But if you're not a gar-dener or these plants don't grow well in your area, buy them from good sources that specialize in local and/or organic herbs. Organic, especially, ensures bet-ter health not only for you but for the planet as well. (See Resources for a list of herb suppliers.)

Herbal Teas

What's the difference between a medicinal tea and a beverage tea? While beverage teas can most certainly be conducive to good health, they are blended and served primarily for plea-sure, with flavor being the guiding fac-tor, rather than the healing properties of the herbs. A medicinal tea, on the other hand, can be flavorful and delicious, but it's blended specifically for health pur-poses. It's a tea blend with a mission. (Of course, the better it tastes, the more compliant the "patient" will be.)

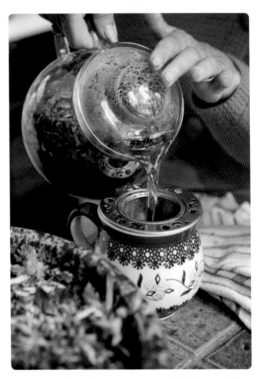

A medicinal tea can be tasty and delicious while also doing its work to ward off an oncoming cold or soothe frazzled nerves.

I seldom direct people to make medicinal teas by the cupful; it is impractical and time consuming. Instead, I recommend making a quart of tea at a time. You can reheat the tea as you need it or drink it at room temperature. Because water doesn't have preservative properties, herb tea doesn't have a long shelf life. Though it'll keep better under refrigeration, it can be kept at room temperature for a day or two, depending on the ambient temperature. But as soon as it starts to taste stale or flat, and/or bubbles start to form, brew a fresh pot.

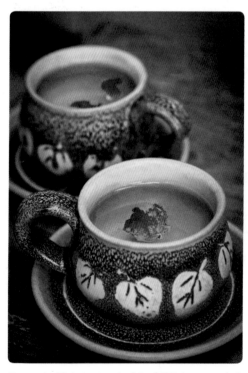

Brewed with intent and a bit of "kitchen magic," herbal tea offers more than meets the eye. Along with herbs and water, there's also earth, sky, sunlight, and stars captured in this cup.

Infusions and Decoctions

When making tea, leaves and flowers are prepared differently from roots and bark, in much the same way that spinach is cooked differently from potatoes. Leaves and flowers are generally steeped in hot water so as not to overcook and destroy the enzymes, vitamins, and precious essential oils. Roots and bark are generally simmered to draw forth the more tenacious plant constituents. There are a few exceptions to these rules, which you'll generally find noted in herb books, including this one. But honestly, if you make a mistake and simmer a root that should have been steamed, don't panic. Your remedy will still work.

The process of steeping a plant in boiling water is called *infusion*, while the process of simmering a plant in lightly boiling water is called *decoction*. When in doubt, steep. Steeping is much less destructive to many of the important medicinal components of plants. The longer you steep the herbs, the stronger the tea. That's not always preferable, as long steeping times can bring out some of the less desirable parts of the plant. Steep black tea too long and what happens? It goes from being a fragrant, aromatic beverage to an astringent-tasting, tannin-rich medicinal tea.

A medicinal tea blend, whether an infusion or a decoction, is defined by its strength and potency. For medicinal purposes, teas need to be fairly strong, and so you'll use a relatively large amount of herbs in making them.

How to Make a Medicinal INFUSION

Infusions are made from the more delicate parts of the plant, such as the leaves, flowers, buds, some berries and seeds, and other aromatic plant parts. Highly aromatic roots such as valerian, ginger, and goldenseal are often steeped rather than decocted, though I find they are effective either way. After, add the spent herbs to your compost. Here are the basic steps.

1. Put 4 to 6 tablespoons of dried herb (or 6 to 8 tablespoons of fresh herb) into a glass quart jar.

2. Pour boiling water over the herbs, filling the jar. Let steep for 30 to 45 minutes. (The length of steeping time and the amount of herb you use will affect the strength of the tea.)

3. Strain and drink.

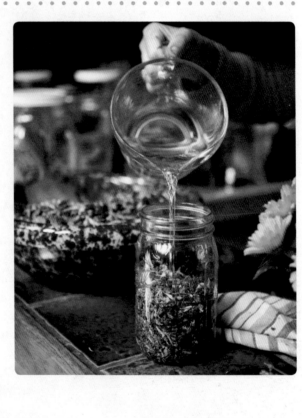

How to Make a Medicinal DECOCTION

Decoctions are made from the more fibrous or woody plant parts, such as the roots and bark, twiggy parts, and some seeds and nuts. It's a little harder to extract the constituents from these tough parts, so a slow simmer is often required. After, add the spent herbs to your compost. Here are the basic steps.

1. Place 4 to 6 tablespoons of dried herb (or 6 to 8 tablespoons of fresh herb) in a small saucepan. Add 1 quart of cold water.

2. With the heat on low, bring the mixture to a slow simmer, cover, and let simmer for 25 to 45 minutes. (The length of simmering time and the amount of herb you use will affect the strength of the tea.) For a stronger decoction, simmer the herbs for 20 to 30 minutes, then pour the mixture into a quart jar and set it aside to infuse overnight.

3. Strain and drink.

Note: *Some people prefer to simmer the tea down to concentrate its properties even further. In this case, smaller dosages will be needed (see pages 46–47 for dosage guidelines).*

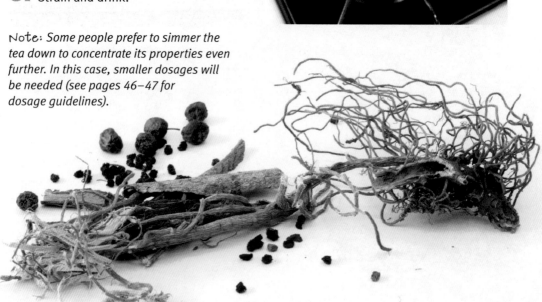

How to Make Solar & Lunar Infusions

Using the light of the sun or moon to extract the healing properties of herbs is one of my favorite methods for making tea. Medicinal teas brewed by this method may not contain the same amount of chemical constituents as those simmered on a stovetop, but they contain a different level of healing that General Electric could never impart.

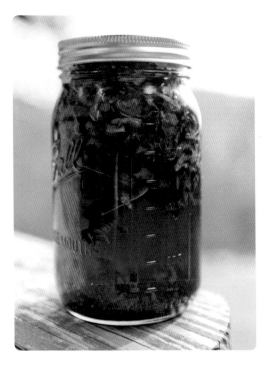

TO MAKE A SOLAR INFUSION, place the herbs (using the same proportions as suggested for infusions and decoctions) in a glass quart jar with a tight-fitting lid. Fill with cold water and cover tightly. Let sit in direct sunlight for several hours.

If you are cold, tea will warm you;
If you are heated, it will cool you;
If you are depressed, it will cheer you;
If you are exhausted, it will calm you.

— WILLIAM GLADSTONE

TO MAKE A LUNAR INFUSION, place the herbs in an open container (unless there are a lot of night-flying bugs around!), fill with water, and position directly in the path of the moonlight. Lunar tea is subtle and magical, and it is whispered that fairies love to drink it. When would a lunar infusion be suitable for healing purposes? Whenever a little extra magic is needed.

Syrups

Once you've learned to make a good medicinal tea, you're two steps away from making syrup. You'll just need to cook down the tea to concentrate it and add sweetener — to sweeten it, yes, but also to preserve it. Our ancestors loved using herbal syrups as medicine not only because they taste delicious, which makes it easier to convince reluctant family members to take their medicine, but also because sugar and other sweeteners are such good preservatives. Visit any of the apothecary sections at living history museums across the country and you'll get a good idea of how important herbal syrups were.

A SIMPLE HONEY-ONION SYRUP FOR COLDS

One of my favorite remedies for colds and sore throats is this very simple, old-fashioned, tasty honey-onion syrup. I learned to make it early on, while living one winter in the "outback" of the Canadian northwest. Far from the neighbors, with a small child in tow, we lived in a little log cabin on the side of the Bugaboo mountain range, relying on our own skills and a certain pervasive spirit of independence that marked the times. The honey-onion syrup simmered on the back of the woodstove, and as we walked by, which we often did, we'd scoop a spoonful into our mouths. I can't remember if any of us got a cold that winter, but if we did, I can bet it was chased away quickly by this hearty syrup.

TO MAKE THE SYRUP: Slice two to four large onions into thin half moons and place the slices in a deep pan. Just barely cover the onion slices with honey. Warm the onions and honey over very low heat, until the onions become soft and somewhat mushy and the honey tastes strongly of onions. You can add chopped garlic, if you want, for an even stronger syrup: stronger medicinally and stronger tasting!

TO USE: Oh, yum. It's actually quite tasty. To help fight off a cold, at the first onset of symptoms take ½ to 1 teaspoon every hour or two. If you already are suffering from a cold, take 1 teaspoon three or four times daily to speed your recovery.

How to Make a Medicinal SYRUP

Children and the elderly seem to prefer syrups, as both age groups are more inclined to down their medicine if it's sweet. "A spoonful of sugar helps the medicine go down" was a ditty most surely written about herbal syrups.

1. Syrups begin with a very concentrated decoction. Combine an herb or herb blend with water in a pot, using 2 ounces of herb per quart of water. Set the pot over low heat, bring to a simmer, cover partially, and simmer the liquid down to about half the original volume.

2. Strain the herbs from the liquid (compost the spent herbs). Measure the volume of the liquid, and then pour it back into the pot.

3. For each pint of liquid, add 1 cup of honey or other sweetener, such as maple syrup, vegetable glycerin, or brown sugar. Most recipes call for 2 cups of sweetener (a 1:1 ratio of sweetener to liquid), but I find that far too sweet for my taste. (Before refrigeration was common, the extra sugar helped preserve the syrup.)

4. Warm the mixture over low heat, stirring well. Most recipes call for cooking the sweetener and tea for 20 to 30 minutes over high heat to thicken the syrup. This certainly does make a thicker syrup, but I'd rather not cook the living enzymes out of the honey, so I warm the mixture only enough that the honey combines with the liquid (not over 110°F; lower is better).

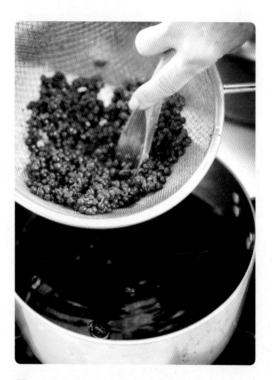

5. Remove from the heat. If you like, add a fruit concentrate for flavor, or a couple of drops of aromatic essential oil such as peppermint or spearmint, or a small amount of brandy to help preserve the syrup and/or to aid as a relaxant in a cough formula.

6. Pour the syrup into bottles. Store in the refrigerator, where it will last for several weeks.

Oils

Have you made garlic oil for salads or mixed flavorful herbs into olive oil for basting your favorite roast? Well, then, you've made herbal oil, which is nothing more than oil infused with herbs. There are a few simple tricks to making really good medicinal herbal oil, such as choosing high-quality oil and getting the temperature just right for extracting the medicinal constituents from the herbs, but it doesn't take long to master the art. And once you've made herbal oil, you're a step away from making salves and ointments.

Choosing Ingredients

By using different combinations of herbs and oils, you can make either strong medicinal oils or sweet-scented massage and bath oils. Though you can use any good-quality vegetable oil, the oil of choice for medicinal oils is olive oil, which is medicinal in its own right, being soothing and rich in oleic, omega-6, and omega-3 fatty acids. Olive oil is also stable, meaning that it doesn't go rancid quickly. It is perhaps not the best oil for bath and body oils, as it tends to be heavy, feels oily, and always smells faintly of olives, but for medicinal oils and salves, there's no finer choice.

The easiest and quickest way to make medicinal oil is the double-boiler method. But I'd also suggest that you try the old-fashioned solar method. There's something about the slow merging of herbal properties into the oil, extracted by that all powerful solar light, that accentuates the qualities of the herbs. There are other methods of making herbal oils as well, but since this is a beginner's guide, let's keep it simple and easy. These two methods work well, are easy to follow, and ensure a good product.

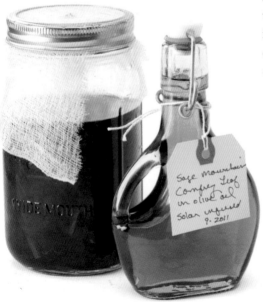

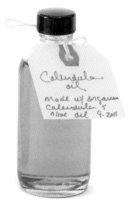

How to Make a Medicinal **OIL**
(Double-Boiler Method)

This quick, simple method makes beautiful oil, as long as you keep the oil at the right temperature. Between 95° and 110°F is perfect.

1. Chop the herbs and put them in the top part of a double boiler. I *strongly* recommend a double boiler instead of a regular pan, as the oil can overheat very quickly, destroying the herbs and oil both. You don't want deep-fried herbs or burned oil, and believe me, either can happen very quickly if you're not using a double boiler.

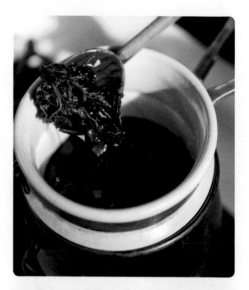

2. Cover the herbs with an inch or two of high-quality cooking oil (preferably olive oil).

3. Slowly bring the oil to a very low simmer, with just a few bubbles rising — no rapid boiling or overheating, please. Simmer gently for 30 to 60 minutes, checking frequently to be sure the oil is not overheating. When the oil looks and smells "herby" — it will become deep green or golden and smell strongly of herbs — then we know the herbal properties have been transferred to the oil. The lower the heat and the longer the infusion, the better the oil.

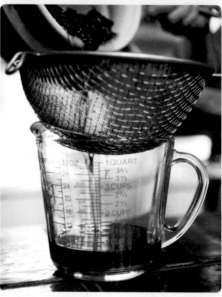

4. Strain out the herbs, using a large stainless-steel strainer, and lined with cheesecloth, if needed. Discard the spent herbs. Let the oil cool, and then bottle and label it. A quick little hint: Don't put the labels on until *after* you have poured the oil and wiped down the outside of the jars, to avoid staining your labels.

How to Make a SOLAR-INFUSED OIL

This, I must admit, is my favorite method for making herbal oils. It uses the great luminary energy of the sun to extract herbal constituents into the oil. How could there not be something healing about that? I learned this method from one of my earliest teachers, Juliette de Bairacli Levy. She would place her jars of herb-infusing oils in sandboxes to concentrate the heat, a technique used in the Mediterranean.

1. Place the herbs in a widemouthed glass jar and cover with an inch or two of high-quality vegetable oil (preferably olive). Cover tightly.

2. Place the jar in a warm, sunny spot and let the mixture steep for 2 weeks.

3. Strain out the herbs, using cheesecloth or muslin. (For a double-strength infusion, add a fresh batch of herbs and infuse for 2 more weeks. This will give you a very potent medicinal oil.) Then bottle the oil.

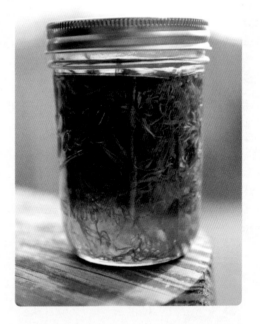

Note: *You can squeeze the last bits of oil from the spent herbs into a separate container. Don't mix this oil with the medicinal herbal oil, as this second straining will most likely have lots of little herb particles in it. You can save this oil for cooking and salad dressings.*

Because oils generally go rancid quite quickly when exposed to heat and light, you would expect these solar-infused oils to spoil within a couple of weeks. However, as long as herbs are infusing in the oils, they don't go rancid. Once poured and strained, they are as susceptible to rancidity as any oil, but during the actual steeping they remain stable. I've never met anyone who could explain this phenomenon to me, so I have to assume it's something to do with the antioxidant properties of the herbs. I do know that this is the way our ancestors made oils, and it has worked wondrously for centuries.

Many people prefer to make oils using fresh herbs, and you certainly can. But I find that high-quality dried herbs, which don't have the water content of fresh herbs, in most cases make a better oil. Water and oil don't mix well; water in herbal oil can introduce moisture and bacteria, which leads to spoilage. When I make oils from fresh herbs, before adding the herbs to the oil, I usually fresh-wilt them: I place them on a basket or screen in a single layer, in a warm area out of direct sunlight, and let them wilt for several hours. They're ready when they look limp. Fresh wilting allows some of the moisture to evaporate, so there's less chance of spoilage.

In general, vegetable oils — other than olive and coconut oils, which are remarkably stable — tend to spoil quickly and don't have a long shelf life. Most oils, if exposed to heat and light, will begin to spoil within a few weeks; unfortunately, many are already rancid when purchased. Rancid oils are a major cause of free-radical damage and related health issues. All oils should be stored in a cool, dark place to prolong their shelf life. Refrigeration is best, but in most kitchens, real estate in the "icebox" is in high demand. So find a place that's cool and dark to store those precious oils. Stored properly, herbal oils made with olive oil will last for several months to a year. When the oil starts to smell "off" or loses its color, it's time to discard it and make a new batch.

What to Watch Out For

Occasionally, condensation will form inside the jar, toward the top. Since water can harbor bacteria in the oil, if this happens, open the jar and use a clean, dry cloth to wipe away the moisture. If condensation is a chronic problem, use a cover of thick layers of cheesecloth, rather than a tight-fitting lid, to allow condensation to evaporate.

If the herbal oil grows mold, there is too much water in the herb or moisture in the jar. Be sure to use dried herbs or to wilt the herbs before using them. Be certain the container is completely dry, and check inside the lid, especially if it has a liner; it often holds moisture.

If your herbal oil starts to smell "off," like rancid butter, don't use it internally or externally. Our skin is our largest organ of assimilation and elimination, and we should treat it well. A bit of healthy advice: If you wouldn't eat it, don't put it on your skin. That sure eliminates a lot of "beauty aids"!

Salves

Once you've made herbal oil, you're a step away from a salve. Salves, also known as ointments, are made of beeswax, herbs, and vegetable oils. The oil acts as a solvent for the medicinal properties of the herbs and provides a healing, emollient base. The beeswax is also a protective, soothing emollient, and it provides the firmness necessary to form the solid salve.

How to Make a Medicinal SALVE

There are a few tricks to making a high-quality salve, but often even the first batch you make will turn out perfectly by following these simple steps.

1. Make a medicinal oil, following the instructions on page 35.

2. For each cup of finished herbal oil, add ¼ cup beeswax. Heat the oil and beeswax together over very low heat, stirring occasionally, until the beeswax has melted. Then do a quick consistency test. Don't skip this step; it's simple, takes only a few minutes, and will ensure that your salve is the thickness you desire. Place 1 tablespoon of the mixture on a plate, then let sit in the freezer for a minute or two. Then check the firmness of the salve. For a harder salve, add more beeswax to the blend. For a softer salve, add more oil.

3. Once the mixture is the consistency you want, remove the blend from the heat and pour immediately into small glass jars or tins. Obviously, you're working with very hot oil, so be careful. This is not a job for children!

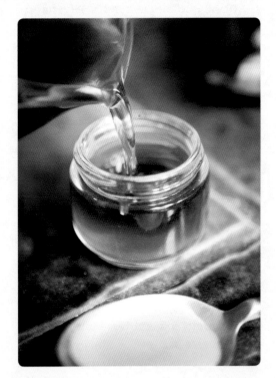

4. Store the salve in a cool, dark place, where it will keep for at least several months. I've had some that lasted for years. (If, however, you keep the salve in a car or in the hot sunlight, it will deteriorate rapidly; the color fades and the oil begins to smell rancid.)

Tinctures

Tinctures, which are very concentrated liquid extracts of herbs, are one of the most popular ways to take herbal medicine internally. They are simple to make and easy to take, and they have a long shelf life. Though I favor medicinal teas for addressing chronic health problems, I appreciate the convenience of tinctures and often recommend them, especially for acute situations. You simply dilute a dropperful or two of the tincture in a small amount of warm water, tea, or juice, and drink. You can take tinctures straight from the bottle as well, but they are rather strong tasting and quite potent.

Most tinctures are made with alcohol as a solvent. Though the actual amount of alcohol you'll consume when taking a tincture is quite small (approximately 1 to 2 teaspoons per day), some people prefer not to use alcohol, and use vegetable glycerin or apple cider vinegar instead. These nonalcohol tinctures are not as potent or strong as the alcohol-based ones, but they do work and are preferred for children and for adults who are sensitive to alcohol.

Choosing a Solvent

If you plan to use alcohol as the solvent for your tinctures, select one that is 80 to 100 proof. "Proof" is a measure of the actual alcohol content of a spirit: half of the proof is the percentage of alcohol in the spirit. For instance, an 80-proof spirit is 40 percent alcohol, and a 100-proof spirit is 50 percent alcohol. The rest of the liquid in the spirit is water. The ratio range of 40:60 (40 percent alcohol and 60 percent water) to 50:50 (50 percent alcohol and 50 percent water) is the perfect medium for extracting most of the properties from herbs, which is why herbalists have used alcohol as a base for herbal medicines for as long as alcohol's been around. It's a perfect pairing. Most vodkas, gins, brandies, and rums are 80 to 100 proof, and any of them will work well in a tincture.

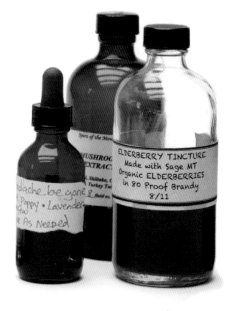

How to Make an Herbal TINCTURE

There are several methods for making tinctures. Though I have run several herbal-medicine companies and can make precisely standardized tinctures, weighing and measuring each ingredient, using fancy equipment, and keeping meticulous records, when I am in my own kitchen, I use the traditional simpler's method (see the box on page 25). It makes as fine a tincture as any made in a lab, and it's so much easier and fun. All that you need to make a tincture with this traditional method are herbs, alcohol (or glycerin or vinegar), and a glass jar with a tight-fitting lid. The herbs can be fresh or dried, but if you're using fresh herbs, you may want to fresh-wilt them first to allow some of the moisture to evaporate.

1. Chop your herbs fine. Place the finely chopped herbs in a clean, dry glass jar.

2. Pour enough alcohol over the herbs to completely cover them by 2 to 3 inches, and then seal the jar with a tight-fitting lid. It's not unusual for the herbs to float to the top. If this happens, let them settle for a day or two, and then check to see if you need to add more alcohol to reach that 2- to 3-inch margin. Sometimes I mark the level of the herbs on the outside of the jar before adding the alcohol, to serve as a guide for how much alcohol to add.

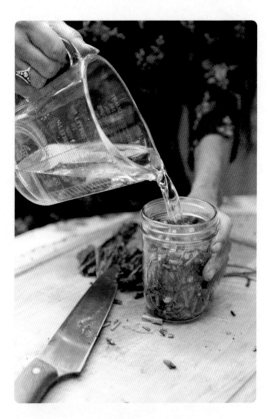

3. Place the jar in a warm, sunny spot, and let the herbs soak (macerate) for 4 to 6 weeks, shaking daily. Is it necessary to shake the bottle daily? It's probably not essential, but I like the idea of infusing my medicine with prayers and healing thoughts every day. On a practical note, shaking allows the solvent to mix thoroughly with the herbs and prevents them from settling on the bottom of the jar.

4. Strain the herbs from the liquid (offer the spent herbs to the compost goddess). Pour the liquid into a clean glass jar with a tight-fitting lid. Store in a cool, dark spot. An alcohol-based tincture will keep for many years, whereas a glycerin tincture will keep for 2 to 3 years and a vinegar-based one at least 1 year, and often much longer.

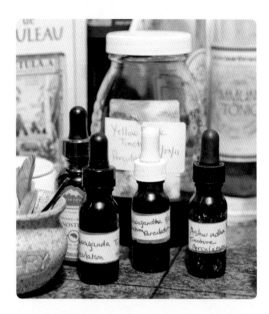

Tinctures are highly concentrated liquid herbal extracts. Easy to make and easy to take, they are among the most popular forms of herbal medicine, but are best diluted in tea, water, or juice.

HOW MUCH IS A DROP?

Tincture dosages are often given in terms of drops or dropperfuls. Here's a quick guide to how much those drops and dropperfuls add up to. (Who was it who counted all those drops? I'd like to thank her!)

TEASPOON MEASURE	DROPPER MEASURE	MILLILITER MEASURE
¼ teaspoon	1 dropperful (35 drops)	1 ml
½ teaspoon	2½ dropperfuls (88 drops)	2.5 ml
1 teaspoon	5 dropperfuls (175 drops)	5 ml

If you're using vinegar as your solvent, warm it before adding it to the herbs to help release the herbal constituents. Remember, vinegar tinctures will not be as strong as alcohol tinctures, as vinegar doesn't break down the constituents as well, nor will it last as long. But vinegar has an advantage in that it's a common culinary substance and can be incorporated into your regular meals (in salad dressing, for example).

Glycerin, a constituent of all animal and vegetable fats, is a sweet, mucilaginous substance that also has solvent properties. It's not nearly as potent as alcohol or as versatile as vinegar, but it has some advantages; primarily, it's very sweet and makes a tasty tincture that children like. Use only food-grade vegetable glycerin for tincturing. It's available in some pharmacies and in most natural food stores. Before adding it to the herbs, dilute the glycerin with water, usually in a ratio of 2 parts glycerin to 1 part water (or more water, if the glycerin is particularly thick).

Herbal Liniments

An herbal liniment is made in *exactly* the same way as a tincture. However, a liniment is used *externally*, while a tincture is generally used internally. Liniments traditionally are used to disinfect cuts and wounds and to soothe sore muscles. There are hundreds of liniment recipes, and I've made a fair number of them. See page 133 for my favorite.

Herbal Pills

Herbal pills are easy to make and practical. You can formulate your own blends and make them taste good enough that even children will eat them. They are excellent for a sore throat; you can formulate them with herbs that fight infection, and sucking on them is by itself soothing to the throat.

Depending on your technique, these little pills can look quite professional. Mine always start off as perfectly round little balls, but eventually, after I tire of rolling, the blend turns into one big glob, which I put in a jar and store in the refrigerator with a small handwritten sign that says ROLL YOUR OWN.

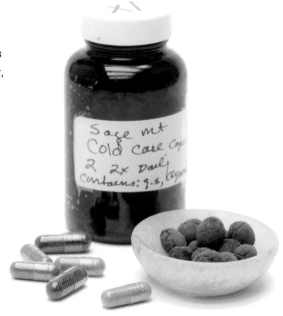

How to Make Herbal **PILLS**

Making herbal pills is a good project to do with children. It's messy, fun, and very easy — and children are more prone to take their medicine if they've had a hand in making it. Carob or cocoa powder is added to make these pill balls tasty as well as effective. Licorice could also be used for this purpose.

1. Place powdered herbs in a bowl and mix with enough water and honey (or maple syrup) to make a sticky paste.

2. If you like, or if the recipe calls for it, add a tiny drop of essential oil to the mixture and mix well. Don't add too much; one or two drops will do. Wintergreen and peppermint essential oils are nice as flavoring agents. Or you might choose other essential oils for the medicinal benefits they'll bring to the remedy.

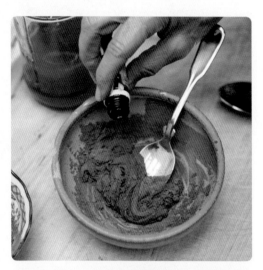

3. Thicken the mixture with enough carob or unsweetened cocoa powder to form a thick, smooth paste. Knead until the dough is as smooth as bread dough.

4. Break off small bits of dough and roll them into small balls, the size of pills. You can roll the pills in carob or cocoa powder for a finished look, if you like.

5. Dry the pills in a dehydrator, or place them on a cookie sheet and dry them in the oven at a very low temperature (around 150°F, or with just the oven light on). If you're having warm, dry weather, you can even sun-dry them.

6. Once dried, these pills will keep indefinitely. Store in glass jars in a cool, dark location.

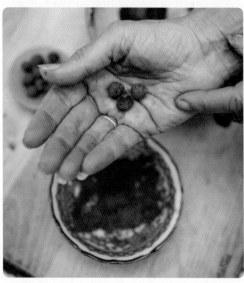

Baths, Poultices, and Compresses

One of my earliest teachers was the great herbalist Juliette de Bairacli Levy. She lived to be almost 100 years old and had a greater impact on modern American herbalism than any other individual. Juliette's success rested in her ability to care, her compassion, her inner knowing and awareness. She relied on the earth's simplest recipes and used plants she found growing nearby, and these she infused with her own touch of wisdom and passion.

Juliette's techniques, too, were simple. She was especially fond of the "laying on of leaves," as she called poultices and compresses, and used them for treating many types of health problems. She also employed cold-water bathing, treating all manner of maladies in the bathtub. Until she was in her late 80s she swam daily, often in the ocean and rivers that were part of the natural landscape around her. Was this daily infusion in the waters of life part of her secret for well-being and rejuvenation?

Following are some of these simple skills or tools that augment or enhance the way herbs work. I'm not convinced that science or modern medicine offers anything quite as practical or effective as these old-fashioned, free-for-the-taking techniques for home health care.

Herbal Bath

WHAT IT DOES: Depending on the herbs you choose and the temperature of the water, you can create a relaxing bath or a stimulating one, a bath that is soothing, or decongesting, or uplifting. Baths open up the pores of the skin, our largest organ of elimination and assimilation. Bathing is nothing less than immersing ourselves in a strong infusion of healing herbal tea. In fact, several prominent healers administer most of their herbal formulas via the bath.

WHAT'S NEEDED: A good old-fashioned clawfoot bathtub is wonderful, but any good-sized tub will do. You'll need herbs, of course, and perhaps essential oils, and you may also want candles and incense. You might as well make this an experience and do it up; it's well worth it!

HOW TO: Place the herbs in a large handkerchief, clean nylon stocking, or strainer and tie it directly to the faucet of the tub. Turn on the water at the hottest temperature, and let the water flow through the herb bag vigorously until the tub is about half full. Adjust the water temperature to a suitable degree; warm to hot is relaxing, cold is stimulating, and tepid is neutral. Finish filling the tub, then add any essential oils.

Poultice

WHAT IT DOES: A poultice is an external application of moist herbs, clay, grated or mashed veggies, or other absorbent material on the skin used to draw out impurities, to soothe, or to increase circulation. Typically a poultice is used to treat insect bites, rashes, burns, sore muscles, sprains, blood poisoning, swollen glands, cysts, boils, pimples, internal injuries, and tumors.

WHAT'S NEEDED: At the most basic level, you'll need herbs and/or whatever other ingredients will be in the poultice. You may want two or three towels or cotton cloths (flannel is my favorite) in which to fold the poultice.

HOW TO: If you're using fresh herbs or vegetables, mash or grate them, and then mix with enough boiling water to form a paste or pulp. If you're using powdered herbs or clay, just add enough boiling water to form a thick paste. Then apply the poultice ingredients to the skin, either directly or folded into a piece of cotton fabric. Cover with a towel. You can keep in the heat by placing a hot-water bottle or heating pad over the poultice. Replace the poultice as it cools down. Repeat as needed, for up to an hour at a time.

Compress

WHAT IT DOES: A compress is an external application of hot or cold liquid on the skin. A hot compress draws blood to the skin's surface, thereby increasing circulation in that area. The heat also pulls impurities to the surface and in some cases can help relieve congestion. A cold compress reduces inflammation and swelling and soothes excess heat, as in cases of sunburn, bruises, strains, sprains, swollen glands, and mastitis.

WHAT'S NEEDED: Soft cotton fabric and hot or cold herbal tea or water.

HOW TO: Prepare a strong herbal tea (usually three times stronger than you would drink). For a cold compress, cool the tea in the refrigerator or by adding ice cubes. For a hot compress, heat the tea on the stovetop, and keep it hot. In either instance, hot or cold, dip a piece of soft cotton fabric in the tea and place directly on the affected area. (For a hot compress, you can place a hot-water bottle or heating pad over the compress to keep it hot and help the heat penetrate the tissues.) Keep the compress on for at least 30, up to 45 minutes, dipping the cloth back in the tea as needed. Repeat several times a day for several days.

Fomentation

WHAT IT DOES: A fomentation is an external application of alternating hot and cold compresses. The fluctuation in temperature causes the capillaries to dilate and constrict. This physical manipulation of blood flow is one of the best and safest mechanisms for removing congestion and obstruction throughout the system.

WHAT'S NEEDED: You'll need two large soft cotton squares and both hot tea (kept hot throughout) and ice-cold water (kept cold with ice cubes).

HOW TO: Apply a hot compress, then leave on for 5 minutes. Next, apply a cold compress, and leave on for 2 to 3 minutes. Repeat, alternating hot and cold, for at least 20 minutes. I've used this process for hours to help people pass gallstones and kidney stones.

The Skinny on Dosage and Duration of Herbal Treatments

Dosage varies according to the size and weight of each person. A basic adult dosage assumes a person of approximately 150 pounds (for children's dosages, see page 48). But other factors play a role in determining the correct dosage, including a person's sensitivity to foods and herbs, overall health, and the particular condition or health issue being treated. One of the most important factors is whether the condition is acute or chronic.

Acute Health Problems

Acute problems are short term, generally come on quickly, have aggressive symptoms, and respond quickly to treatment; examples are toothache, headache, fever, nausea, stomach distress, menstrual cramps, cuts, scrapes, and wounds.

Pharmaceutical medications are generally very effective for relieving acute symptoms. They are designed to get rid of symptoms quickly — sometimes to the detriment of the system as a whole. Herbal remedies also work well for acute situations, but they don't always have as dramatic an effect.

For example, upon noticing the early symptoms of a cold coming on, you could perhaps avert the illness by taking ½ teaspoon of echinacea tincture every hour. But if you took the amount of echinacea tincture often recommended on the bottle (30 drops two times daily), you'd most likely still end up with that

DOSAGE FOR ACUTE HEALTH PROBLEMS

Because the situation is active and symptomatic, it's necessary for the remedy to work quickly and efficiently. The point is to see symptoms improve quickly. Generally, small dosages given frequently are more effective than large dosages taken over longer periods of time. As a guideline, dosages are:

- ¼ cup of herbal tea every half hour, for a total of up to 4 cups per day

- ½ to 1 teaspoon of herbal syrup every 2 hours, for a total of up to 10 teaspoons daily

- ¼ to ½ teaspoon of herbal tincture every hour, for a total of up to 6 teaspoons daily

- 1 or 2 herbal capsules or pills every 2 hours, for a total of up to 8 capsules daily

darn cold; a smaller dosage taken much more frequently would be more effective.

As another example, to address a raging fever, rather than drinking 1 cup of fever-reducing tea (with, say, yarrow, peppermint, and elderberry) three times a day, you might drink ¼ cup every half hour, until the fever subsided.

Chronic Health Problems

Chronic conditions usually develop over a period of time, often arise because of lifestyle choices and/or genetic factors, and are generally more challenging to treat. Because they are long term, they usually require a longer period of treatment. Herbalists often say, for every year you've had a chronic problem, you'll need a month of treatment to heal it. For example, if you've had allergies for 6 years, plan on following an herbal program for 6 months. That's arbitrary, of course, but the point is that there's no quick fix for chronic issues. Herbal and other natural therapies are ideal for treating chronic problems because they address the foundational or core issues that cause the problems while modifying or eliminating the symptoms. Pharmaceutical medications, on the other hand, generally address only the symptoms. While they can be quite effective for relieving the symptoms of a chronic problem, they often make the actual problem worse.

Take breaks from the herbal program, not because the herbs will build up and/or have toxic side effects, but because it's always good to give your system a break. Relax, skip the dosages for a day or two each week you're following the program, then resume and continue.

DOSAGE FOR CHRONIC HEALTH PROBLEMS

If a chronic problem is causing acute symptoms, often you'll need to treat those symptoms using the dosages recommended for acute problems. But for long-term treatment of the foundational issue(s), it is better to give larger doses over a longer period of time. Most often, the key to success in addressing chronic problems is consistency: remembering to follow the program and take your herbal remedies for the designated period of time.

As a guideline, dosages are:

- 3 to 4 cups of herbal tea daily
- 1 to 2 tablespoons of herbal syrup twice daily, or as needed
- ½ to 1 teaspoon of tincture two or three times daily, for a total of up to 3 teaspoons daily
- 2 or 3 capsules or pills two or three times daily, for a total of up to 6 capsules daily

USING HERBS TO TREAT CHILDREN

People are often wary of treating children with herbs, and they might treat themselves with herbal remedies but opt to give pharmaceuticals to their children because "the doctor says so." This seems odd and contrary, as herbal remedies are generally so much safer and children respond quite well to them. It's up to parents, of course, to decide what they feel is best for their own children. But a quick look at the side effects of even the safest over-the-counter medications for children and a similar look at the herbs used for children's health might convince them of the safety and efficacy of using herbal remedies, especially for those simple, common issues we address in this book.

Suggested Dosages for Children

When adult dosage is 1 cup (8 ounces)	
AGE	DOSAGE
Younger than 2 years	½ to 1 teaspoon
2 to 4 years	2 teaspoons
4 to 7 years	1 tablespoon
7 to 12 years	2 tablespoons

When adult dosage is 1 teaspoon	
AGE	DOSAGE
Younger than 3 months	2 drops
3 to 6 months	3 drops
6 to 9 months	4 drops
9 to 12 months	5 drops
12 to 18 months	7 drops
18 to 24 months	8 drops
2 to 3 years	10 drops
3 to 4 years	12 drops
4 to 6 years	15 drops
6 to 9 years	24 drops
9 to 12 years	30 drops

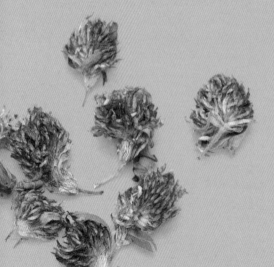

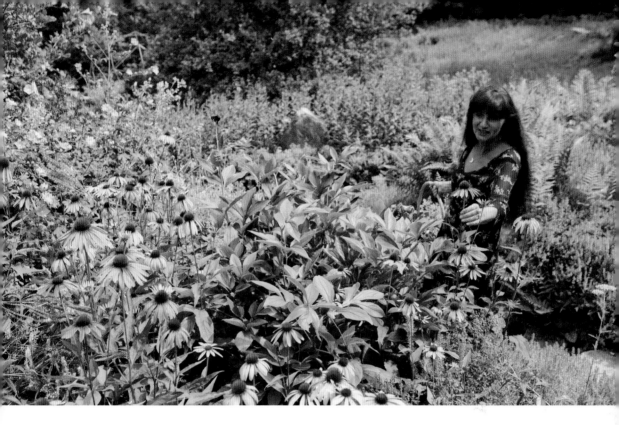

Congratulations!

You've done it — completed Herbal Medicine Making 101. Celebrate by moving over the outdated medications that usually fill people's medicine cabinets and stocking up on fresh herbal products, products you've made yourself, using ingredients you know are fresh and nonharmful. Try using these products when you or your family members come down with a cold, cough, sore throat, and any of the other common ailments that we humans are known to get. If your homemade remedies aren't as effective as you'd like them to be, or you're not getting as well as quickly as you'd expect, you can always scoot down to the local drugstore. And, of course, call a professional health-care practitioner whenever it seems necessary.

There are no fixed methods to apply to the human predicament, there is no single all-pervasive rule to follow, since medicine is not a science but an art.

— MICHAEL MOORE, *herbalist & author*

CHAPTER 3

9 Familiar Herbs & Spices to Grow and Use

THE HERB AND SPICE CABINET contains a marvelous cornucopia of medicinal plants. Most people are unaware that the herbs and spices they sprinkle on their food are renowned healing agents, respected through the ages by manifold cultures. Almost every one of these common culinary heroes makes wonderfully effective kitchen medicine. There's been many a time when I've been visiting friends or family and heard someone complain of a cold or flu or headache. Though my hosts may not have a home apothecary filled with medicinal herbs or an herb shop close by, I can confidently open their spice cabinet and find in there what I need to make an effective herbal remedy. People sometimes think I have some kind of special "magic," but I'm just doing what our ancestors have always done.

Though we tend to associate the flavor of certain herbs with certain foods — basil with tomatoes, cloves with meat, horseradish with hearty meat dishes — often these pairings came about for medicinal reasons, not flavor. Basil aids with the digestion of the acids in tomatoes; cloves and other spices helped preserve meat in prerefrigeration days; and horseradish stimulates sluggish digestion and aids in the digestion of fatty foods. Indeed, in this way many medicinal plants have entered into the household via the kitchen door, ushered in by the Mistress of Spices, their healing spirits camouflaged in culinary garb.

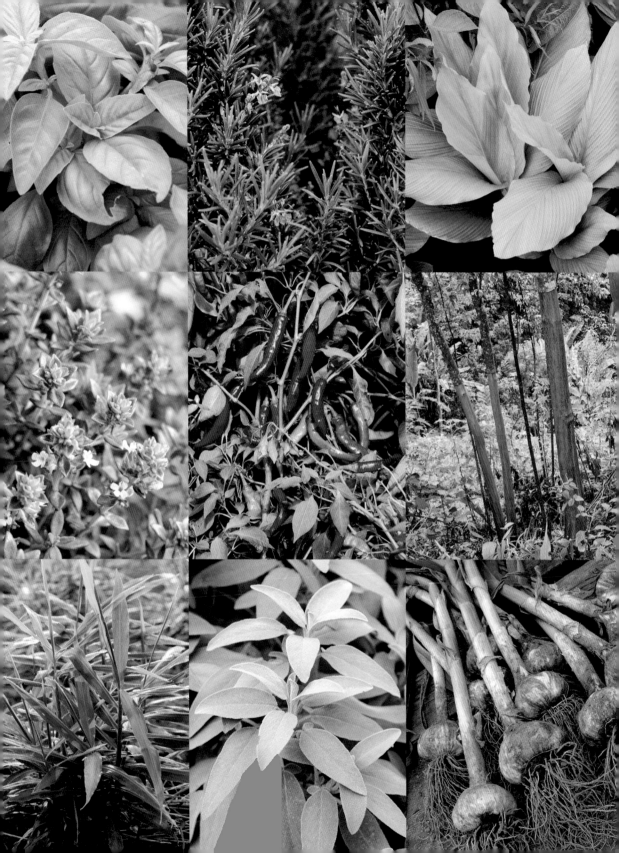

WHEN IS AN HERB MEDICINE AND NOT FOOD?

There's wisdom in that old adage *Let food be your medicine and medicine your food*. Truly, it's the diet and lifestyle choices we make on a daily basis that most affect our long-term health and well-being. It's odd that *health care* becomes an issue only when health is absent, and *medicine* is deemed effective only if it's so potent that the possible side effects are often as serious as the initial diagnosis. Health care really makes more sense if we care enough about our health to attend to it on a regular basis, and medicine makes more sense if it's strong enough to be effective but still kind to our bodies. Always start with the most effective but least harmful remedy. Isn't the healer's primary creed *First, do no harm*?

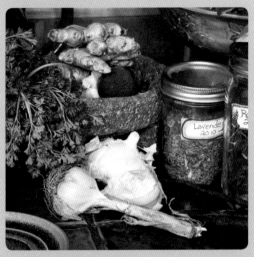

A combination of garlic, parsley, and fresh ginger morphs from food to medicine as a result of how it's prepared and the dosage amount.

As you'll learn in this chapter, many of the herbs, spices, and foods you eat daily are considered medicines. So what's the difference between a medicine and a food? The difference lies primarily in the dose, duration, and preparation. For instance, a cup of fresh-juiced carrot, beet, and dandelion root with ginger is a delicious pick-me-up tonic. Drinking a cup of this tonic now and then is going to make anyone feel energized. But for this same tonic to be an effective *medicine* used to treat a specific condition, such as liver congestion, poor digestion, and/or recurring skin problems, you would need to drink 2 to 3 cups of this blend daily for 2 to 3 weeks. The occasional cup of ginger tea is delicious and may even be helpful for relieving menstrual cramps. But to be used medicinally, with effective and lasting results, a woman would need to drink small amounts of it throughout the days of her menstrual cycle. Garlic used occasionally in your cooking may help support overall heart health, but to lower cholesterol and treat a circulatory condition, you'd need to take a specific amount of garlic on a regular basis.

In this way, dosage, duration, and preparation morph a culinary herb into a powerful medicinal remedy.

Basil / *Ocimum basilicum*

With over 150 varieties grown around the world, basil is renowned for its distinctive flavor, scent, essential oil, and healing properties. The kind typically found in the kitchen is sweet basil, *Ocimum basilicum*. Its genus name, *Ocimum*, derives from the ancient Greek word for "smell"; its species name, *basilicum*, is also of Greek origin and means "kingly" or "royal herb." Indeed, basil was once used in salves prepared for royalty. Also valued by us common folk, basil has enjoyed an enduring popularity in both the kitchen and the apothecary.

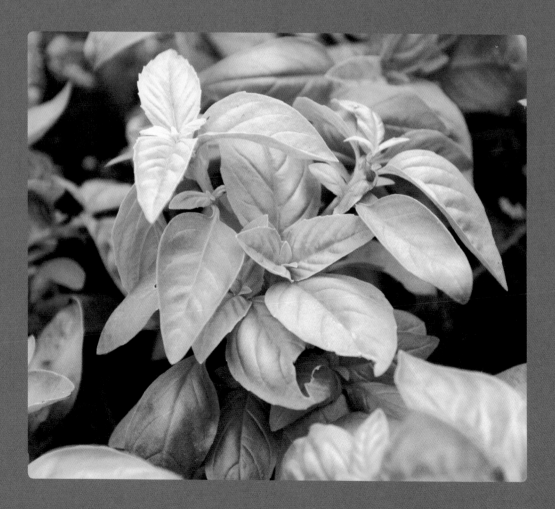

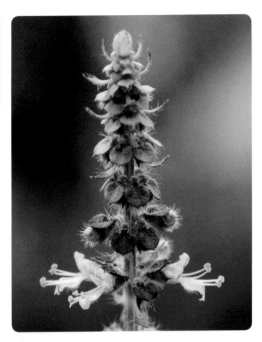

Basil reigns supreme in the garden and is renowned for its distinctive flavor, scent, essential oil, and wonderful culinary and medicinal uses.

Parts used

Leaf and flowering top

Key constituents

Essential oil, caffeic acid, monoterpenes, tannins, beta-carotene, vitamin C

Safety factor

Completely safe, tried and true; no known side effects. Use freely and abundantly.

GROWING BASIL

Sweet basil is an annual, easy to grow but sensitive to cold weather. Seeds can be sown directly in the soil after temperatures have warmed to at least 50°F. Or sow seeds indoors in flats to get an early start. These are sun-loving, warm-weather plants, so grow them in fertile soil in full sun. Set or thin the plants to 6 to 8 inches apart. The secret to healthy, bushy plants loaded with beautiful leaves is to keep them well fertilized during the growing season with fish emulsion or manure tea. Pinch off the flowers to prevent the plants from becoming "leggy" and to ensure a long season of growth. To harvest, pick leaves as they mature throughout the entire season. Six to eight plants should provide you with fresh basil throughout the season and enough for pesto and vinegars for the winter months as well.

MEDICINAL USES

Sweet basil acts principally on the digestive and nervous systems, easing gas and stomach cramps and preventing or relieving nausea and vomiting. It is mildly sedative and has been found to be helpful in treating nervous irritability and fatigue, depression, anxiety, and insomnia. It also has antibacterial properties, and the juice or a poultice of the fresh leaves relieves the itch and pain of insect bites and stings.

Basil Poultice

I have found a basil poultice to be quite effective in relieving the sting and swelling of mosquito and other insect bites.

To make the poultice:
Mash and/or chew a handful of fresh leaves until soft.

To use:
Place the leaves directly on the insect bite or sting. Leave on for 15 to 20 minutes. Repeat as necessary, until the swelling and itching are relieved.

Variations

* If fresh leaves are unavailable, rehydrate a few dried leaves with enough water to make a mash, and apply.

* For an even more effective remedy, prepare a poultice using equal parts fresh basil leaves and fresh plantain leaves.

Basil Tea for Headache & Stress

You can use either fresh or dried herbs for this tea blend.

>> 1 part basil leaf
>> 1 part lemon balm leaf
>> ¼ part chamomile and/or lavender flower

To make the tea:
Combine the herbs and mix well. Use 1 teaspoon (if dried) or 2 teaspoons (if fresh) of the herb blend per cup of boiling water. Pour the boiling water over the herbs, let infuse for 10 to 15 minutes, then strain.

To use:
Drink warm or at room temperature. Headaches are always helped by soaking your feet in hot water (as hot as you can stand). Even better, add a drop or two of lavender essential oil to the footbath. And better yet, have a friend quietly rub the nape of your neck and your shoulders. . . . Sit back, sip your tea, soak your feet, and feel your headache drift away.

Medicinal Basil Pesto

A pesto is simply an herb paste. Though few rival the flavor of a classic pesto made with all the yummy goodness of fresh basil, pine nuts, Parmesan, garlic, and olive oil, pestos can combine basil with other medicinal herbs. Depending on the herbs you use, you can pack a powerful punch of nutrients and healing factors into a delicious and nutritious pesto without your family ever suspecting they are "taking their medicine." Any combination of medicinal plants will work, depending on the desired effect. For cleansing heavy metals and toxicity from the body, for example, you could use the following:

» ½–1 cup olive oil

» 1–3 cloves garlic

» 1 cup fresh cilantro leaves and stems

» ½ cup fresh basil leaves

» ½ cup fresh dandelion leaves

» ½–1 cup pine nuts or walnuts

» ¼ cup freshly grated Parmesan, Pecorino, or other hard cheese

To make the pesto:
Combine the olive oil, garlic, and fresh greens in a blender or food processor. Pulse until smooth.

Add the nuts and cheese and pulse again, until the mixture reaches the desired consistency (I prefer my pesto a little chunky, rather than creamy smooth).

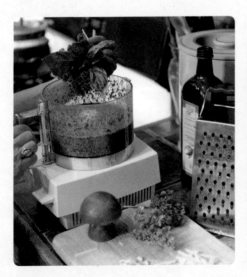
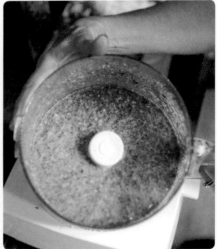

To use:

Pesto can be enjoyed on just about anything — crackers, grains, pasta, soup — or even by itself! Even when it's made with medicinal plants, the flavors seem to blend and harmonize into something sublime. It's medicine at its finest: it tastes good, is easy to make, and is a very efficient way of getting lots of nutrient-dense medicinal plants into your diet.

Make and freeze enough medicinal (and culinary) pesto blends so you'll have them available through the winter months. Unless you're lucky or smart enough to live in an area where fresh herbs grow year-round, you won't be able to make these pestos once summer's over, so plan ahead.

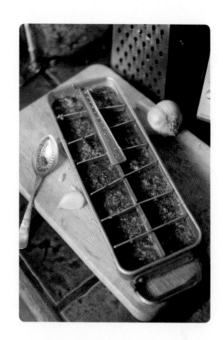

. . . .

Variations

You can use this basic recipe to make any number of medicinal herb pestos. The proportions will vary, depending on personal taste and intention (the desired effect). Try mixing 1 cup wild herbs with 1 cup common culinary herbs. Taste as you go — some of these herbs are suprisingly strong, but good! Some good pesto herbs are the following:

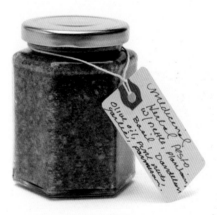

Wild Herbs

* Amaranth
* Chickweed
* Lamb's-quarter
* Nettle
* Plantain

Culinary Herbs

* Marjoram
* Mint
* Oregano
* Sage
* Thyme

Holy Basil / *Ocimum sanctum*

I really couldn't have a discussion about basil without mentioning holy basil, or tulsi, as it is commonly called. Holy basil (*Ocimum sanctum*) grows wild throughout India. It is one of the most highly regarded herbs in that country and has more than 3,000 years of recorded medicinal use. In Ayurvedic medicine, India's widely practiced healing system, holy basil is classified as a *rasayana*, an herb that nourishes a person's growth to perfect health and promotes long life. The daily use of this herb is believed to help maintain the balance of chakras, or energy centers in the body, and to bring out the goodness, virtue, and joy in humans. Bring out the tulsi!

Holy basil and sweet basil share similar medicinal qualities and are often classified together, but they have some different properties as well. Holy basil is an excellent adaptogenic tonic herb that helps restore vitality and vigor. Sweet basil may have these qualities as well, but it more

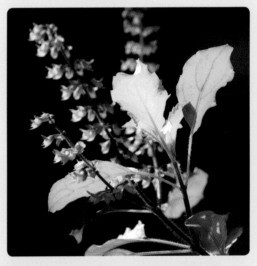

specifically addresses imbalances and illnesses; you might say that it is more medicinal and specific in its action. You can use one in place of the other, but as you use them you'll discover their differences. I generally choose sweet basil for treating headaches and digestive disturbances and holy basil for restoring vitality and renewing energy.

Holy Basil Tincture

For stronger medicine, tincture fresh holy basil.

To make the tincture:
Follow the instructions for making holy basil vinegar, but use 80-proof alcohol instead. (See page 40 for more-detailed instructions for making herbal tinctures.)

To use:
Take ½ to 1 teaspoon of the tincture two or three times daily as a rejuvenating adaptogenic tonic.

Holy Basil Long-Life Vinegar

Making delicious vinegar with fresh holy basil is a great way to enjoy this herb daily. For vinegars I usually suggest using raw, unpasteurized apple cider vinegar. It is rich in nutrients and active enzymes, it is alkalinizing to the system, and it helps establish healthy gut flora, the bacteria that live in our digestive tract and are essential to good health. If you want to make herbal vinegar for culinary purposes, you can use wine vinegar, but for medicinal purposes, there's no substitute for apple cider vinegar.

To make the vinegar:

Pack a clean widemouthed quart jar about three-quarters full with holy basil leaves. If necessary, wash the leaves first and gently pat dry. Fill the jar nearly full with raw, unpasteurized apple cider vinegar. Put on the lid and shake gently a few times.

Set the jar in a warm, sunny window or by a heat source and let steep for 3 to 4 weeks, until the vinegar takes on the rich, pungent taste and odor of the herb. For a double-strong vinegar, discard the spent herbs and repeat the process.

When the vinegar is ready, strain and rebottle, perhaps in a fancy old vinegar bottle or wine bottle. (You wouldn't want to steep the herbs in such a bottle, though; trying to fish spent herbs out of a narrow-necked bottle is time-consuming and sometimes downright impossible!) If you like, add a sprig or two of fresh herb to the finished product for a visual touch.

To use:

Drizzle 2 to 3 tablespoons of vinegar over your daily salad. Or drink a small toddy of it (¼ cup or less) daily. Or blend it into a veggie drink for a quick pick-me-up and a lively flavor.

Variations

Of course you can get creative with your holy basil vinegar, adding all kinds of tasty herbs to enhance the flavor and medicinal properties. Try adding garlic cloves, whole cayenne peppers, or sprigs of rosemary, sage, or thyme. There's no end to the creative fun you can have in your kitchen apothecary lab!

Because of its legendary curative properties, its exciting flavor, and its magical ability to sustain a sense of well-being, cayenne is one of my favorite herbs for both medicinal and culinary purposes. An herb supreme for warming the system, cayenne gets blood circulating through cold fingers, toes, and other extremities and gives an overall sense of warmth. It's an excellent analgesic, often used topically to relieve pain. And no herb works better to relieve congestion. I couldn't imagine getting through a winter without it.

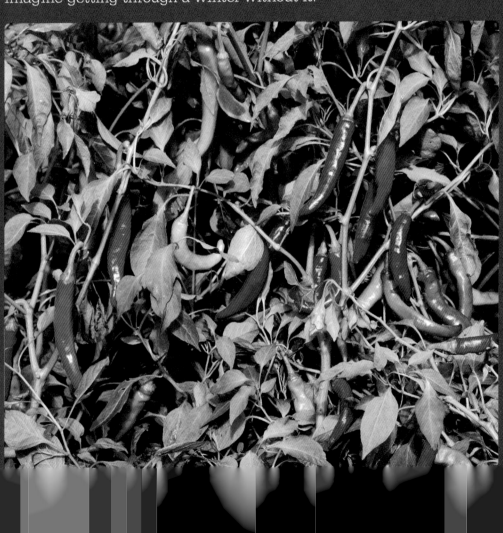

GROWING CAYENNE

Cayenne is fairly easy to grow. An annual, it does best with a long growing season, warm weather, fertile soil, and full sun. But it's tolerant. It thrives even in my own northern Vermont, which is perhaps less well suited for growing cayenne than other places, and after a good summer (more sunshine than rain) we're able to harvest a host of little bright red chiles.

MEDICINAL USES

Cayenne is a warming circulatory stimulant, a safe and effective tonic for the heart, and an excellent digestive aid. One of its active ingredients, capsaicin, stimulates circulation throughout the body and assists in digestion by stimulating the release of both saliva and stomach enzymes. Capsaicin also signals the brain to release endorphins, the body's "feel-good" hormones. And capsaicin has proved so effective as a topical pain reliever for arthritis, bursitis, and muscle and joint aches that it's the active ingredient in several over-the-counter pain-relief creams. Rich in vitamins A and C, cayenne can aid and support the immune system, which is one of the reasons it's so useful in formulas for colds and flus. Cayenne also has a long history of use as a heart herb. Dr. John Christopher, a well-known and much-beloved herbalist of the mid-twentieth century, recommended it both as first aid for a heart attack and as a tonic to strengthen the heart. Recent scientific studies done in the United States and India show that cayenne lowers cholesterol and may help reduce the severity of heart disease.

Part used

Only the fruit is edible and medicinal. As is the case for other members of the Solanaceae (nightshade) family, to which cayenne belongs, the leaves, stems, and flowers can be toxic.

Key constituents

Capsaicin, carotenoids, vitamin C, flavonoids, steroidal saponins, volatile oils

Safety factors

Cayenne, though perfectly safe, needs a warning sign: This herb is hot! If for no other reason, you should use it cautiously. When handled directly, compounds in the chile can burn the skin, especially for those who have fair or sensitive skin; if that's the case for you, wear gloves when working with cayenne. Don't touch your eyes after handling cayenne, as it will sting. Cayenne is a strong stimulant and can cause stomach convulsions if taken in large amounts. The most important thing is to use appropriate dosages. Small amounts go a long way with this herb.

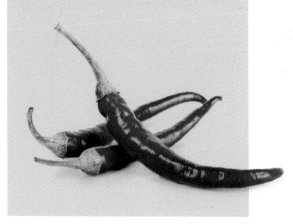

Cold Care Capsules

One of my favorite recipes for keeping a cold at bay or getting over one more quickly, these Cold Care Capsules are easy to make but pack a big punch. Take the half hour or so that's required to make a batch, and keep it on hand for the cold season. You can find gelatin or vegetable capsules at most herb shops and natural foods stores, and some pharmacies.

» 1 part echinacea root powder

» 1 part goldenseal root powder (organically cultivated)

» ½ part marsh mallow root powder

» ¼–½ part cayenne powder (depending on your heat-tolerance level)

» "00" gelatin or vegetable capsules

To make the capsules:

Mix the powders together in a small bowl. Scoop the powder into each end of a capsule, packing tight, and recap. It takes only a few minutes to cap 50 to 75 capsules, a winter's worth for most families. Store in a glass jar with a tight-fitting lid.

To use:

At the first sign of a cold or flu coming on, take 2 capsules every 2 to 3 hours until the symptoms subside, or up to 9 capsules a day. This is a high dose and should not be continued for longer than 2 to 3 days, at which time you should decrease the dose to 2 capsules three times a day (the normal adult dose for most herbal capsules; see pages 46–47 for further information on appropriate dosages).

THE CAPSULE MACHINE

If you plan to make a lot of capsules, a handy little device called the Capsule Machine will shorten the job and might be a worthy investment (it runs about $15). It's made by a company called Capsule Connection and is available from many herb shops and online.

SIZZLING FOOT WARMER

Cayenne is an effective circulatory herb for those who have poor circulation and is a popular remedy for warming cold hands and feet. Try sprinkling a small amount of cayenne (no more than 1/8 teaspoon) in your shoes to help warm your toes. If you find cayenne alone to be too hot or irritating, mix it with an equal amount of dried ginger powder.

Creaky Bones Cayenne Rub

This salve is excellent for soothing achy joints and creaky bones. Be careful not to touch your eyes or other "delicate parts" after using it, though, and wash your hands well.

» ½ cup olive or peanut oil
» 1 tablespoon cayenne powder or flakes
» ⅛ cup beeswax
» A few drops wintergreen essential oil

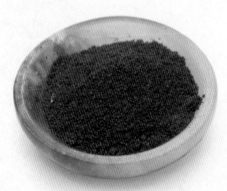

To make the salve:
Following the instructions on page 35, make an herbal oil with the oil and cayenne. (It will be difficult to strain out the cayenne powder, so just let it settle to the bottom and try to leave it there.) Use the herbal oil and the beeswax to make a salve, following the instructions on page 38. After removing the salve from the heat, add enough wintergreen essential oil to scent the salve sufficiently; it should have a strong but not overbearing smell. Pour into jars.

To use:
Rub a fingerful or so over aches and pains to soothe and relieve.

Cinnamon / *Cinnamomum verum*

Cinnamon is a familiar kitchen spice around the world, adding fragrance and warmth to everything from breakfast cereal and cookies to curries and roasts. But what most people don't realize is that cinnamon is also a potent, powerful, well-researched medicine.

Cinnamon is actually the bark of fast-growing trees, members of the laurel family, native to Sri Lanka and India. The bark is harvested from young shoots that sprout from the stumps of the trees, which are cut back every couple of years. The bark is high in essential oils, coumarins, tannins, and other chemical constituents that help define its medicinal uses.

Cassia (*Cinnamomum cassia*), a close relative of cinnamon, is native to China, where it is used much like its cousin in medicinal and edible preparations. However, cassia tends to be warmer, more fragrant, and stronger tasting. But the two can be and often are used interchangeably.

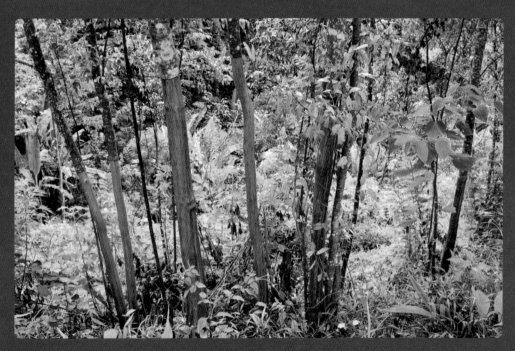

GROWING CINNAMON

A tropical native, cinnamon prefers warm, moist conditions and sandy soil. Depending on the variety, it matures as either a large tree or a large shrub and definitely will require a large space in the garden. North America generally does not offer the best growing conditions for cinnamon, and it is not commonly grown here. But if you happen to live in a particularly warm, moist region and have a large backyard, why not be the first person in the neighborhood to grow your very own cinnamon?

MEDICINAL USES

Because of its warming and stimulating properties, cinnamon is used to boost vitality, improve circulation, and clear congestion. It is a well-respected digestive aid, particularly for cases of overeating, bloating, and sluggish digestion, and one of the best herbs around for stabilizing blood sugar levels. It is also a powerful antiseptic, with antiviral and antifungal properties, and is often indicated in cases of viral infections, fungal infections, and colds and flus. It is a mild emmenagogue, making it useful in cases of sluggish and painful menstruation. And finally, because of its sweet, warming flavor, cinnamon is often used in medicinal formulas simply to improve their flavor.

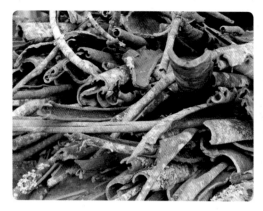

What we know as cinnamon stick is actually the inner bark of young plant shoots.

Part used

Inner bark of the tree (powdered, chopped, or as whole sticks)

Key constituents

Essential oils, tannins, iron, magnesium, mucilage, zinc, coumarins

Safety factor

Though cinnamon is generally considered safe and nontoxic (have you ever seen a warning label on a spice jar in the supermarket?), it does have slight emmenagogic properties (meaning it stimulates the uterus); while it may be useful to help encourage a late menstrual flow, it's not recommended in large amounts in the early stages of pregnancy. (Truthfully, though, there aren't any reports of a miscarriage resulting from the use of cinnamon.)

Cinnamon-Ashwagandha Rejuvenating Milk

The herb ashwagandha is commonly used in Ayurvedic medicine to promote peaceful sleep and as a potent rejuvenating tonic. This warm milk, made with ashwaghandha and cinnamon and sweetened with a touch of honey, is a delicious and nutritive drink, especially useful in the evening for those who have trouble relaxing or falling asleep.

» 1 cup milk (cow, almond, Rice, or any other)

» 1 teaspoon ashwagandha powder

» 1 teaspoon cinnamon powder

» 1 teaspoon honey (or to taste)

To make the milk:
Warm the milk, then add the powders and honey. Stir well, taste, and adjust the flavors if necessary.

To use:
Pour into a cup and drink slowly a couple of hours before bedtime.

Cinnamon-Ginger Tea for Menstrual Difficulties

Both cinnamon and ginger are reliable aids for relieving stomach and menstrual cramps. A warm poultice or hot-water bottle placed over the pelvic area can also be helpful.

» 1 teaspoon chopped cinnamon baRK

» 1 teaspoon chopped dried ginger or freshly grated gingerroot

» Honey, as desired

To make the tea:
Pour 1 cup boiling water over the herbs. Cover and let steep for 30 to 45 minutes. Strain, and sweeten with honey if desired.

To use:
Sip slowly. Prepare and drink as often as needed, until cramps subside.

Cinnamon Honey

I'm not sure how "medicinal" this honey really is, but there's no question that it's delicious. You can use as much or as little cinnamon as you want, depending on the strength you prefer.

» ½ cup honey
» 1–2 tablespoons cinnamon powder

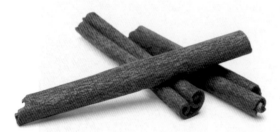

To make the honey:
Gently warm the honey until it is stirrable, and then stir in the cinnamon.

To use:
Stir a teaspoon of the honey into warm water or herb tea. Or spread it over buttered toast. Or just lick it off a spoon; it's that delicious!

Cinnamon Tincture for Stabilizing Blood Sugar

If you are troubled by either high or low blood sugar, try this tasty remedy. In concert with a healthy diet, plenty of exercise, and reduction in stress levels, cinnamon can be extremely helpful in regulating blood sugar.

» 2–4 ounces chopped cinnamon bark
» 80-proof alcohol (brandy, vodka, or gin)

To make the tincture:
Place the cinnamon in a widemouthed glass quart jar. Cover with 2 to 3 inches of alcohol. Let steep for 4 to 6 weeks, shaking daily. Strain through a fine-mesh, stainless-steel strainer lined with cheesecloth. Discard the cinnamon, then bottle the liquid.

To use:
Take ¼ to ½ teaspoon two times a day for 5 days. Take 2 days off, then repeat the cycle. Continue in this manner for several weeks, or until blood sugar levels normalize.

Warming Cinnamon Bath Salts

Bathe in cinnamon? Why not? Cinnamon is warming, decongesting, antiseptic, and antiviral and is a wonderful aid for colds and congestion. Any sea salt will do, but use large Celtic salt grains if you can find them, as they add more minerals to the bathwater.

» 3 tablespoons cinnamon powder

» 1 tablespoon gingerroot powder (optional)

» 1 cup sea salt

To make the bath salts:
Stir the powdered herbs into the salt. Store in a sealed glass container.

To use:
Add ¼ cup of the bath salts to a bathtub filled with warm water. Stir well and step in.

Variation

Not exactly medicinal, but certainly healthy, sensuous rose-cinnamon-cardamom bath salts are especially lovely for a romantic evening.

» 3 tablespoons cinnamon powder

» 1 tablespoon cardamom powder

» ¼ cup rose petals

» 1 cup celtic salt (unrefined and chunky is nice)

» 5–10 drops cinnamon essential oil (optional)

» 5–10 drops cardamom essential oil (optional)

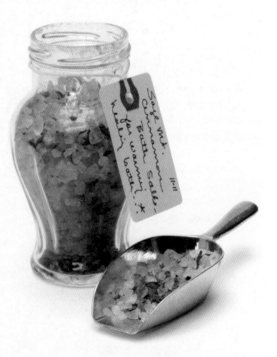

Cinnamon Spice Chai

A delicious tea blend that originated in India, chai has as many recipes as drinkers. Here's one of my favorite chai recipes. Use it as a warming, energizing tea in the morning, or ice it for a cool afternoon pick-me-up.

» 1 part chopped cinnamon bark

» ½ part coriander seed

» ½ part chopped gingerroot

» ¼ part coarsely ground black peppercorns

» ¼ part cracked cardamom seeds (put in herb mill and grind quickly)

» ⅛ part whole cloves

» Darjeeling tea (or your own favorite black or green tea)

» Honey (to taste)

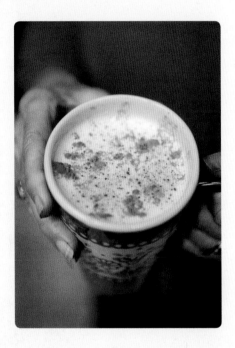

To make the chai:
Combine the cinnamon, coriander, ginger, peppercorns, cardamom, and cloves and mix well. Using 1 teaspoon of the herb mixture per cup of water, simmer the spices for 15 to 25 minutes. Remove from the heat, add an appropriate amount of Darjeeling (depending on how many servings you've brewed), cover, and let steep 5 minutes. Strain, then sweeten to taste with honey.

To use:
Drink! I love this tea with frothed milk. It rivals the best latte and offers so much more in health-giving properties.

Garlic / *Allium sativum*

Were I forced to have only one herb in my kitchen, garlic would
be it. If there's anything that enhances the flavor of food more or
improves health better than garlic, it's yet to be discovered. Garlic,
the infamous stinking rose, brunt of many jokes, offender of probing
proboscises, may, in the final analysis, be nothing less than one of
the world's most versatile culinary herbs and greatest medicinal
plants. "Useful for everything" is my motto for garlic.

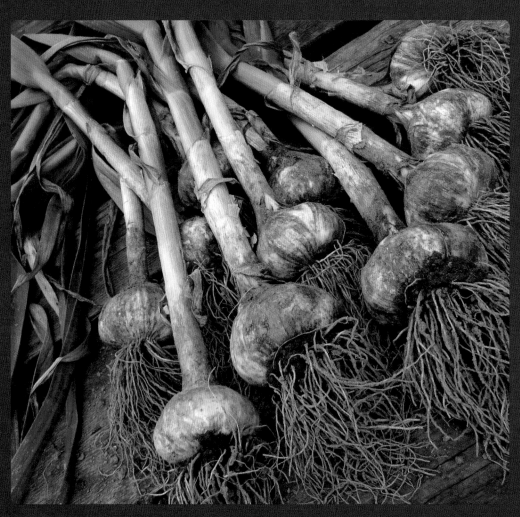

GROWING GARLIC

Garlic is easy and fun to grow. It thrives in well-drained, fertile soil with a good pH (4.5 to 8.5) and does best in full sun. Plant individual cloves with their pointed ends up about 6 inches apart and 2 inches deep. Plant in the fall for a late-summer harvest or early spring for a late-fall harvest. Harvest the bulbs after the blooms die back and the leaves begin to fall over. To increase the size of the bulbs, cut back the flowering stalks, known as scapes. (The scapes themselves are edible and delicious.) Oh, yes, and remember to save some of your biggest, best cloves for replanting.

MEDICINAL USES

Garlic is the herb of choice for treating colds, flus, sore throats, and poor or sluggish digestion. It stimulates the production of white blood cells, boosting the body's immune function, and its sulfur compounds and essential oils make it a potent internal and external antiseptic, antibacterial, and antimicrobial agent effective for treating many types of infections. It has even been found effective against several forms of antibiotic-resistant strains of bacteria. Garlic is also a well-known vermifuge and is used to treat intestinal worms in humans and animals. It is very effective for maintaining healthy blood cholesterol levels and helps prevent blood platelet aggregation, making it the herb of choice for many circulatory issues. Studies show that it also lowers blood sugar levels, making it a useful aid in treating type 2 diabetes. Aside from all this, garlic is just plain tasty.

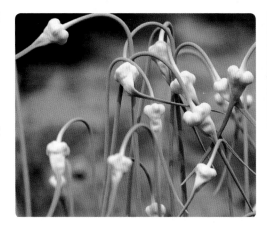

Garlic scapes are lovely in the garden, add interest to bouquets, and make flavorful additions to pesto, soups, and stir-fries.

Parts used

Bulb and scape

Key constituents

Alliin (which converts to allicin when the bulbs are crushed), essential oils, sulfur compounds, germanium, selenium, potassium, magnesium, phosphorus, vitamin A, B vitamins, vitamin C

Safety factors

Yes, garlic does come with warnings. Though generally considered a safe, nontoxic herb, garlic is not necessarily good for everyone. For some, garlic can add too much "fire" to the system, causing heartburn or stomach distress, and sometimes even provoking anger (considered a "hot" condition). Garlic can be a stomach irritant for small children and infants; it should be avoided by nursing mothers who find after eating garlic that their child becomes fussy or colicky. Also, garlic can irritate and burn sensitive skin if applied topically.

Pickled Garlic

Another of my favorite "medicinal" recipes. I learned to make pickled garlic from an old-timer who used to visit my first herb store, Rosemary's Garden, back in the early 1970s. He'd bring in little jars of pickled garlic that he imported from China for me to sell at my shop (when things from China were still a novelty). But they were quite expensive, and I thought it would be far less expensive to make them myself. And it was!

To pickle the garlic:
Fill a widemouthed glass jar with whole peeled garlic cloves. Add enough tamari and/or apple cider vinegar (preferably unpasteurized) to completely cover the garlic. Place the jar in a warm spot (near a sunny window is fine) and let sit for 3 to 4 weeks.

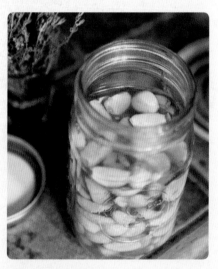

These tasty morsels of pickled garlic contain all the medicinal properties of fresh garlic.

Strain off the liquid. Set half of the liquid aside to be used in salad dressings and marinades. Place the rest of the liquid in a saucepan and add an equal amount of honey. Warm over very low heat, stirring, until the honey is thoroughly mixed into the tamari or vinegar. Pour this sauce back over the garlic, recap, and let sit another 3 to 4 weeks. Store in a cool, dark location, where it will keep for a year or longer — though it never lasts that long, as it's so good!

To use:
Eat at will! Pickled garlic is quite delicious, with a sweet, hot, pungent flavor. This is a great way to eat raw garlic with all of its virtues intact, without fear of the stomach distress that raw garlic is known to sometimes cause.

Without garlic, life would be plain boring.

Four Thieves Vinegar

There are many recipes for this famous vinegar. Here's my own.

» 4 cloves garlic, finely chopped

» ½ cup lavender flowers

» ½ cup rosemary leaves

» ½ cup sage leaves, coarsely chopped

» ¼ cup thyme leaves

» 1 teaspoon clove powder

» Apple cider vinegar (preferably unpasteurized)

To make the vinegar:
Place the garlic and herbs in a widemouthed glass quart jar and add enough warmed apple cider vinegar to cover them. (Warming the vinegar allows it to more actively draw the properties out of the herbs.)

Place the jar in a warm spot (near a sunny window is fine) and let sit for 3 to 4 weeks. Strain, then pour into a glass jar with a tight-fitting lid. Store in a cool, dark location, where it will keep for up to a year.

To use:
According to sources from antiquity, you can use Four Thieves Vinegar to protect against the spell of sorceresses, to ward off the plague, and for endurance and protection — basically the same things you'd use it for today, in a language of a different time. Take 1 to 2 tablespoons every 3 to 4 hours to ward off illness, and use liberally as a flavoring agent.

RAW VS. COOKED

According to the latest studies, cooking garlic may render it a bit less potent, but most of its active ingredients will remain active. So add garlic freely to soups, casseroles, pastas, and other culinary recipes. For complete medicinal benefits, eat it raw, by blending it with pesto (see recipe, page 56) and other sauces. Or try the delicious recipe for Pickled Garlic on page 72.

Fire Cider

This is my favorite herbal vinegar. It's an amazingly effective remedy for staying healthy in the winter and keeping colds and flu at bay. It's actually delicious! Use it as a salad dressing, but be sure to save some for medicinal purposes.

» 1 medium onion, chopped

» 4–5 cloves garlic, coarsely chopped

» 3–4 tablespoons freshly grated gingerroot

» 3–4 tablespoons freshly grated horseradish root

» Apple cider vinegar (preferably unpasteurized)

» Honey

» Cayenne powder

To make the vinegar:
Combine the onion, garlic, ginger, and horseradish in a widemouthed glass quart jar and add enough warmed apple cider vinegar to cover them. (Warming the vinegar allows it to more actively draw the properties out of the herbs.) Place in a warm spot (near a sunny window is fine) and let sit for 3 to 4 weeks. Strain, then discard the spent herbs. Now the fun part: Add honey and cayenne *to taste*. The finished product should taste lively, hot, pungent, and sweet.

To use:
Take 1 to 2 tablespoons at the first sign of a cold, and repeat the dose every 3 to 4 hours until symptoms subside.

GARLIC BREATH?

If you want to avoid garlic breath, try eating a few springs of parsley with your garlic. Or chew anise, fennel, or dill seeds after a garlic-rich meal or a dose of garlic medicine. A small drop of peppermint oil mixed in ½ cup warm water not only will freshen your mouth and aid digestion after a meal, but also help dispel the rich garlic aroma. But the best "remedy" of all for garlic breath is getting others to eat it with you!

Garlic Herb Oil

Another way to eat garlic as "medicine" that is tasty and healing. Mixing garlic with oil makes it less irritating for people with sensitive digestion.

» Several cloves garlic, chopped

» Rosemary, thyme, and oregano leaves (or an herb blend of your choice)

» Olive oil

To make the oil:
Combine the garlic and several teaspoons of herbs in a small pan. Add just enough olive oil to cover the them by an inch or two. Warm over very low heat for 30 minutes, or until the oil tastes strongly of herbs. You can strain the herbs out if you want, but I don't; I love their crunchy texture and flavor in the oil. Pour the oil into a glass jar with a tight-fitting lid. Store in a cool, dark location, where it will keep for several weeks, or in the refrigerator, where it will keep for months.

To use:
Garlic herb oil can be used in many ways: as a spread for bread or crackers, added to soups, or tossed over pasta or rice. Remember, food is the best medicine! The more we can include medicinal herbs as part of our daily diet, the healthier we'll be.

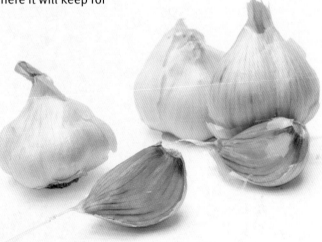

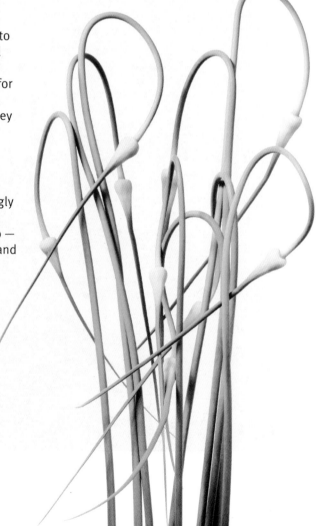

Garlic Flower Oil

Often people toss garlic's lovely scapes and flowering tops, not realizing what a culinary wonder they are, or that they are also medicinal. Scapes and flowers contain much of the same medicinal properties as the bulb, albeit in less potent quantities. If you find garlic bulbs to be difficult to digest or too strong for your taste, try the scapes and flowers. (Use only the tender tops of the scapes, as the bottom part can be quite tough.) Scapes and flowers are lovely additions to stir-fries, imparting a delicious garlicky flavor. We enjoy them best blended in pesto or preserved in olive oil, as I'll describe here.

To make the oil:

Fill a glass jar with chopped garlic scapes and flowering tops. Fill the jar with olive oil. Let sit in a warm place for 2 to 3 weeks. Then move to a cool, dark spot, where the oil will keep for several weeks, or store in the refrigerator, where it will keep for several months. Don't remove the scapes and flowers from the oil; they are tender and delicious.

To use:

This oil can be used in the same way as Garlic Herb Oil (see recipe, page 75), but it isn't quite as strongly flavored. Spread on toast, use as a sauce on rice or pasta, add to soup — just don't waste the garlic scapes and flowers!

Garlic Ear Oil

This is the remedy that I used on my own children and grandchildren when they would, as children do, wake up with an ear infection. I learned it from my grandmother, who, I'm sure, learned it from her grandmother. Hopefully, my grandchildren will remember and pass it on to their grandchildren. It is truly one of the best remedies for ear infections associated with colds and respiratory congestion. (It is not effective and shouldn't be used for "swimmer's ear" and other instances where the infection is caused by water entering the ear.) The garlic fights the infection, and the warm oil is soothing and helps relieve the pain. Of course, if the ear infection doesn't improve with the garlic oil treatment within 24 hours, or if it gets worse, a trip to your family health-care provider is in order. Quickly. Don't let ear infections go untreated, as they can result in a perforated eardrum and permanent hearing loss.

» 1–2 cloves garlic, peeled and sliced

» 2 tablespoons olive oil

To make the oil:
Combine the garlic and olive oil in the top of a double boiler. Warm over very low heat for 10 to 15 minutes, or until the oil smells strongly of garlic. Use a stainless-steel strainer lined with cheesecloth to strain out the garlic. Strain well; *no* garlic pieces, no matter how tiny, should be left in the oil. Pour the strained oil into a small glass dropper bottle. Store in a cool pantry or closet, where the oil will keep for several weeks, or in the refrigerator, where it will keep for several months.

To use:
Each time you use the oil, it needs to be warmed; just place the dropper bottle in a pan of hot water until the oil is, say, the warmth of mother's milk. Be sure the oil is *warm*, not hot. If in doubt, do a test drop in your own ear.

Dispense a dropperful of the warm garlic oil down each ear. The ear canals are connected and the infection can move back and forth, so always treat both ears. If possible, hold a warm, dry cloth over the ears after applying the oil, and/or gently massage around the ears. Repeat every 30 minutes, or as needed until pain subsides.

Another of our kitchen medicine miracles, ginger runs a close second to garlic in versatility and popularity, both culinarily and medicinally. It's a tasty remedy, so people are more willing to use it. I often mix ginger with less tasty medicinals to make them more appealing. And ginger is highly regarded as a medicinal herb. It's an effective remedy for cramps, nausea, morning sickness, and motion sickness. When they were teenagers, my twin daughters found it quite effective for the occasional menstrual cramps they would experience, and they soon turned their friends onto it; hot ginger honey tea was a favorite remedy at Spalding High. While I can generally convince my husband to try anything, he's especially fond of Hot Ginger Balls (see page 82), which he uses ardently to calm the motion sickness that often plagues him when he's deep-sea fishing. Ginger is also wonderfully warming and decongesting; hot ginger tea with lemon and honey and a couple of Cold Care Capsules (see page 62) is often all it takes to activate the immune system.

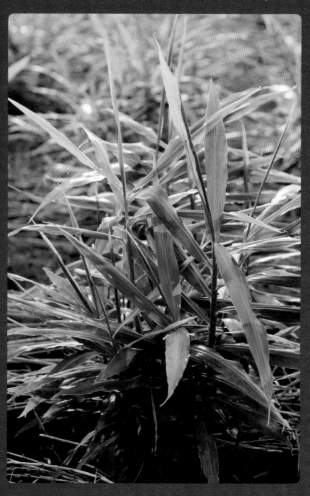

GROWING GINGER

Ginger, a native of Asia, thrives in hot, humid environments in rich, moist soil. I grow ginger year-round in my sunroom, usually starting it from ginger that has sprouted in my kitchen, but the plant goes dormant in the cooler, drier winter temperatures.

Plant pieces of the rhizome with a growing nub or two attached just under the soil. Don't plant deeply or the rhizome will rot. Water frequently, keep the soil moist, give it plenty of sunshine, and your ginger will thrive. Generally, rhizomes are ready to harvest in 8 to 10 months.

Please note: There is a "wild ginger" native to North America, known as *Asarum canadense*. Though medicinal as well, *Asarum canadense* is much stronger and can be toxic if used in large amounts. It is *not* a replacement for true ginger, *Zingiber officinale*. Don't confuse the two; they are entirely different genera.

MEDICINAL USES

Ginger contains a proteolytic enzyme that has been shown to reduce inflammation and help repair damaged joints and cartilage tissue; no wonder it's been a longtime favorite for treating arthritis and joint pain. It improves circulation in the pelvis and is often a main ingredient in reproductive tonics for men and women and in formulas for menstrual cramps and PMS. Numerous studies confirm that ginger lowers blood-level triglycerides linked to diabetes and heart disease. And several clinical studies find ginger more effective than over-the-counter medications for nausea, motion sickness, and seasickness (something every herbalist knows). Clinical studies also show that ginger rivals antinausea drugs for chemotherapy, without their side effects. Its antiseptic properties make ginger highly effective for treating gastrointestinal infections, and it is used in formulas for food poisoning. It is a popular warming, decongesting herb used for cold-type imbalances such as poor circulation, colds and flus, respiratory congestion, and sore throat. All this and it's delicious, too!

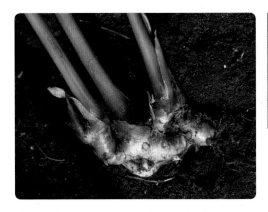

Versatile and tasty, the large fleshy rhizome of ginger is both a culinary delight and effective medicine for a variety of common illnesses.

Part used

Rhizome

Key constituents

Essential oils, oleoresin, gingerol (an acrid constituent that gives ginger its hot taste and stimulating action)

Safety factor

A popular culinary herb used by millions of people, ginger has no known negative side effects.

Ginger Lemon-Aide

This is a fabulous herbal remedy for cramps, colds, congestion, and fevers. You can use bottled lemon juice, but because it's been heated in the bottling process, much of what's good about lemons has been cooked out. I use bottled lemon juice occasionally for cooking when I'm in a hurry or don't have lemons on hand, but for medicinal purposes, fresh lemons are the way to go.

» 4-6 tablespoons freshly grated gingerroot

» 1-2 lemons

» Honey (to taste)

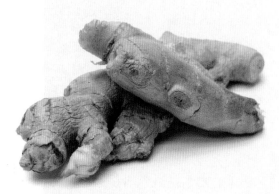

To make Ginger Lemon-Aide:
Combine the ginger with 1 quart cold water in a saucepan. Cover the pan tightly and bring just to a boil. Remove from the heat and let steep 10 to 15 minutes. While the ginger is steeping, squeeze the juice from one or two lemons. Strain the ginger from the tea, if you like, and then stir in the lemon juice and honey to taste for the finishing touch.

To use:
Drink warm or hot.

Variation

For medicinal purposes, it's best to drink Ginger Lemon-Aide hot or warm, but you can also make a delicious summer fizzle from this basic recipe. Make a strong ginger infusion as directed above, using just 2 cups of cold water. Add lemon juice and honey, then refrigerate to cool. Just before serving, add an equal amount of sparkling water.

Ginger Syrup

Years ago, when I was eager to make everything by hand, at home, and healthier than what I could buy at the store, I decided to make candied ginger using honey instead of sugar. Well, it didn't work, of course, as honey doesn't solidify like sugar, but I ended up with the most delicious ginger herbal syrup, and I've been making it ever since. It is a very tasty remedy for motion sickness and stomach distress, colds, coughs, overeating, and other maladies, as well as being a sweet treat on toast.

To make the syrup:

Peel a large hand of fresh gingerroot, then grate it and put it in a pan. Add just just enough honey to barely cover the ginger. Simmer over low heat for 10 to 15 minutes, until the ginger is soft and mushy and the honey tastes strongly of ginger. You can strain the ginger from the honey if you dare, but it's generally a mess, as honey doesn't strain easily. I just leave the ginger in the syrup, as it's soft and adds texture and flavor. Pour the ginger syrup into a glass jar. Refrigerated, it will last for several weeks.

To use:

Use 1 tablespoon as needed for a cold, stomach cramps, and menstrual discomfort. Or add 2 to 3 tablespoons to 1 cup hot water for hot ginger tea.

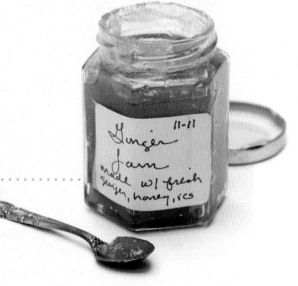

Variation

I've made a simple ginger jam from this recipe. While the syrup is still warm, pour it into a blender. Add 1 to 2 tablespoons of arrowroot powder or cornstarch for each cup of syrup, as a thickener, and blend, which turns the mixture into a delicious ginger jam.

Hot Ginger Balls (a.K.a. Hot Balls)

» 2 tablespoons gingerroot powder

» 1-2 tablespoons carob or unsweetened cocoa powder

» 1 tablespoon cinnamon powder

» Honey

To make the balls:
Combine the ginger, carob or cocoa powder, and cinnamon in a bowl, then mix in enough honey so that the mixture takes on the texture of bread dough. Add ½ teaspoon water, mix well, and knead for a few minutes. (Add more ginger powder or carob or cocoa powder to thicken if necessary.)

Roll into pea-size balls. Let dry at room temperature or in a dehydrator, and store in a glass jar with a tight-fitting lid. Kept in a cool, dark location, these little balls will keep for 3 to 4 weeks; they'll keep even longer if stored in the refrigerator.

To use:
Take two or three balls as needed to calm an upset stomach. For motion- or seasickness, take two or three balls an hour before traveling, so they have a chance to start working, then take as needed.

Hot Ginger Poultice

This is an old-time remedy for relieving menstrual cramps and stomach tension.

To prepare the poultice:
Bring a kettle of water to a boil. Prepare a poultice of ginger using ½ cup of freshly grated gingerroot or 4 to 6 tablespoons of powdered ginger mixed with enough boiling water to make a thick paste. Soak a dishcloth with boiling water, then place the ginger on the hot cloth, folding the cloth over it. Let cool just enough so that it won't burn the skin.

To use:
Apply the poultice directly over the pelvis or stomach area. Keep the poultice hot by placing a hot-water bottle over it. Leave in place for 15 to 20 minutes, or until cramps subside. This remedy is most effective when served with hot Ginger Lemon-Aide (see page 80).

Rosemary / *Rosmarinus officinalis*

I must admit, I have some preference for this herb, as it is my namesake. I'm named after my two grandmothers, Mary Egitkanoff on my mother's side and Rose Karr on my father's side, and the name seemed to stick and grow with me, or I with it. In any case, under the careful guidance of my grandmother Mary, I followed in her herbal footsteps.

Rosemary, the herb, is native to the Mediterranean, grows freely in much of southern Europe, and is cultivated throughout the world. Its genus name, *Rosmarinus*, means "dew of the sea," in reference to the plant's natural habitat on the warm, sunny hillsides bordering the sea.

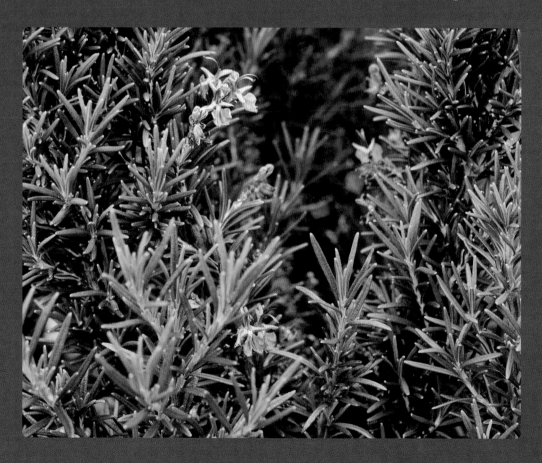

GROWING ROSEMARY

I grew up surrounded by the large rosemary bushes that thrived in the warm, sunny California farmland of my childhood. Since moving to Vermont, I've become a rosemary murderer. Rosemary can't survive freezing temperatures, and so where I live now, it must be brought indoors for a good part of the year. It detests dry heat (many of us in New England heat with wood), strongly dislikes having its feet wet (don't overwater) but doesn't like being dried out either (don't underwater), needs full sunshine (which means it will demand the sunniest window of the house), and loves breezes (keep the fan going or else powdery mildew will develop). But aside from that, it's "easy" to grow!

I've figured out how to keep my rosemary plants healthy at last, but only after killing nearly a dozen fine specimens. Here's what I've learned: A rosemary plant is best cultivated from a root cutting or stem layering. It loves fertile soil and full sunlight, though it will tolerate some shade. Water thoroughly, and don't let the soil dry out completely between waterings, but don't overwater either. To have a really happy rosemary plant, mist the leaves weekly with a diluted seaweed spray. Rosemary planted outdoors (it does well in Zones 7 to 10) can live to be quite elderly, so give it a place in the garden where it can thrive for many years. It can stand a little cold weather but generally will need to be covered and/or brought in if temperatures dip below 40°F, though some hardy plants can withstand colder temperatures. Trim back any dead branches. We often cut back rosemary plants quite severely (removing one-third of the tops) in the late fall before bringing them in for the winter.

MEDICINAL USES

Rosemary is a legendary brain tonic, improving concentration and memory. It enhances the cellular uptake of oxygen and is a mild and uplifting stimulant, and it has long been valued for its ability to ease headaches and migraines and relieve mild to moderate depression. It is also a well-known circulatory stimulant, useful for problems associated with the cardiovascular system, poor circulation, and low blood pressure.

Research shows that rosemary contains high levels of rosmaricine, which acts as a mild analgesic, and antioxidants, which together make it useful for treating inflammation, such as in arthritis and joint damage. Whether used fresh or dried, it is a good digestive aid, facilitating the digestion of fats and starches.

Parts used

Leaf and essential oil

Key constituents

Flavonoids, rosmarinic acid, essential oil, tannins, resin, bitters, camphors, beta-carotene, vitamin C, calcium, iron, magnesium, triterpenes

Safety factor

Rosemary has a long recorded history of use and few reports of toxicity or side effects.

Rosemary-Lemon Thyme Tea

This is a deliciously refreshing, mildly stimulating tea. Lemon thyme is one of the nicest thymes for tea, but of course if you don't have it, any other thyme will do. Or try growing some lemon thyme yourself!

To make the tea:
Prepare an infusion of rosemary and lemon thyme, following the instructions on page 29. Add a teaspoon of lemon juice and a touch of honey, if you'd like.

To use:
Drink as you please.

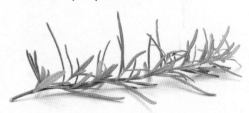

Brain Tonic Tincture

Among the most famous of all my herbal tincture recipes. I've had many students report that they see improvement in their memory within 3 to 4 weeks of beginning this tincture regimen.

» 1 part ginkgo leaf
» 1 part gotu kola leaf
» ½ part rosemary leaf
» ¼ part peppermint leaf
» Brandy

To make the tincture:
Prepare a tincture with the herbs and brandy, following the instructions on page 40.

To use:
Take ½ to 1 teaspoon three times a day for 3 to 4 weeks. Results may be subtle, but generally after 2 to 3 weeks people notice they have better name recall, they remember where they put a list, and even start recalling what was on the list.

Note: *Ginkgo can be contraindicated for people who have problems with heavy bleeding: that is, during menstruation and/or when cut or wounded. It should not be taken for 2 weeks before and after surgery.*

Sage / *Salvia officinalis*

There's an old adage that where rosemary thrives in the garden, the woman rules the house, but where sage thrives, the man rules. Perhaps there's some truth to it; my rosemary thrives, but sage seems to shrivel in my gardens. Woe be to the man who loves me!

Sage is another remarkable culinary remedy, as valuable in the medicine cabinet as in kitchen. I've used sage for all manner of home remedies over the years, from my famed Good Gargle for a Bad Throat to remedies for hot flashes in menopausal women, for uncomfortable night sweats in men, and for nursing mothers ready to wean their toddlers. It's one of those safe, easy-to-use, readily available remedies. Most people have sage in the garden or in their kitchen cupboard, waiting for that one big meal of the year when it's brought forth to stuff the bird. How unfortunate that such a great herbal remedy is so often ignored.

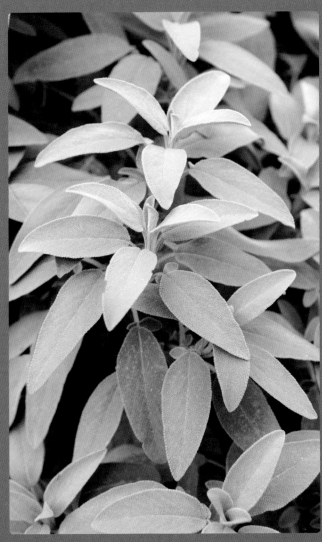

GROWING SAGE

There are more than 750 salvias around the world, and though many varieties are medicinal, the one we'll discuss herein is common garden sage (*Salvia officinalis*), which is hardy in Zones 4 to 8. Garden sage is an easy-to-grow perennial, given the right conditions. It loves full sunshine, warm to hot conditions, and well-drained soil. It doesn't do well in wet or soggy soil and soon tires of cool, wet weather. It's difficult to start from seed, so get your plants from a nursery or propagate them from root cuttings. Older plants will get leggy and woody, so cut back old growth in the early spring, before new growth starts.

Part used

Leaf

Key constituents

Camphor, thujone, cineole, flavonoids, phenolic acids (including rosmarinic acid), tannins, bitters

Safety factors

Sage can affect the quantity of a nursing mother's milk; if used daily (1 cup or more of tea a day), it will decrease the flow of milk substantially. So, obviously, a nursing mother should avoid it, unless she wants to dry up her milk. Although sage contains very little thujone (said to be the active ingredient in absinthe), thujone can be toxic. For this reason David Hoffman, author of *Medical Herbalism*, recommends no more than 15 grams of sage leaf per dose. Also, sage can cause indigestion in certain individuals.

MEDICINAL USES

Sage is a superb aid in the digestion of rich, fatty meat. It also helps lowers cholesterol levels and is a bitter tonic for the liver. It is an excellent herb for rebuilding vitality and strength during long-term illness. Sage tea is a warming, bracing drink, nice mixed with mint or rosemary and lemon balm for a tasty stress reliever.

Sage is a mild hormonal stimulant and can be effective in promoting regular menstruation, offering relief from hot flashes and night sweats. Sage is also helpful for men who have issues with premature ejaculation or "night emissions," a funny term for a quite troubling problem. It is also an effective remedy for leukorrhea, a common vaginal infection. Sage seems to work, in part, by "drying" and regulating fluids in the body. It helps reduce sweating and is often an ingredient in deodorants. It is an old-time but remarkably effective remedy for "drying up" mother's milk; it's so effective, in fact, that nursing mothers are told not to eat or drink much of it. It has been used to mitigate excessive saliva production in those with Parkinson's disease.

Sage is a well-known cold and flu fighter. Because of its astringent, antiseptic, and relaxing action on the mucous membranes, sage is the classic remedy for inflammation of the mouth, throat, and tonsils. It is one of the best remedies for laryngitis, tonsillitis, and sore throat, as a spray or gargle, and it can be used as a mouthwash or swab to treat infected or sore gums and canker sores.

Good Gargle for a Bad Throat

This is an effective gargle for a sore throat. It doesn't taste particularly good, but it works so darn well that it's easy to get people hooked on it.

» 1 tablespoon dried sage leaves

» 1-2 tablespoons salt

» 1 teaspoon goldenseal root powder (organically cultivated)

» A pinch of cayenne powder (optional)

» ½ cup apple cider vinegar (preferably unpasteurized)

To make the gargle:

Pour ½ cup boiling water over the dried sage. Cover and let steep for 30 to 45 minutes, then strain. Add the salt, goldenseal powder, and cayenne, if using, to the still-warm tea and stir to dissolve. Stir in the apple cider vinegar.

To use:

Gargle a teaspoon or two of this mix every ½ to 1 hour. The longer you can stand to gargle, the better. Don't swallow; it won't be harmful, necessarily, but it sure won't taste good.

Sage Mouth & Throat Spray

Tastier than a gargle, this sage spray might be more popular with your less herbally inclined friends, though it may not be quite as effective. For more healing power, replace the brandy with 1–2 tablespoons echinacea tincture.

» 2-3 tablespoons dried or fresh sage leaves

» ¼ cup brandy or vodka

» 1-2 drops peppermint essential oil

» 1 tablespoon honey (optional) for its soothing and sweetening properties

To make the spray:

Pour 1 cup boiling water over the sage. Cover and let steep for 30 minutes, then strain. Drink ¼ cup. Combine the remaining ¾ cup with the brandy or vodka, the peppermint essential oil, and the honey, if using. Store in a bottle with a mister or spray top.

To use:

Spray directly in your mouth as often as needed.

Antioxidant Herb Sprinkle

Sprinkle this blend on any favorite dish: grains, pasta, salads, eggs, veggie drinks. I've used it on virtually everything but desserts!

>> Dulse (seaweed) flakes
>> Dried Rosemary leaves
>> Dried parsley leaves
>> Dried sage leaves
>> Dried thyme leaves
>> Toasted sesame seeds

To make the herb blend:
Combine the herbs in equal proportions, or whatever proportions best suit your own taste.

To use:
Sprinkle away! If you want to add salt, use a coarsely ground Celtic salt, black Hawaiian salt, or pink Himalayan salt. A pinch of cayenne powder or coarsely ground black pepper will give it some zip. Dried nettles, dandelion greens, and plantain leaves are other tasty additions.

Sage Pesto

This is a great recipe for a healthy, healing herb paste. Sage dominates the flavor of this pungent, strong pesto. You can use less sage if you find it overpowering. Of course, if you have fresh wild herbs such as dandelion greens, chickweed, and plantain, add those as well for their healing nutrients.

>> ½ cup fresh cilantro leaves
>> ½ cup fresh parsley leaves
>> ¼–½ cup fresh sage leaves
>> 2–3 cloves garlic
>> ¾–1 cup olive oil
>> ¼–½ cup sunflower seeds (or walnuts, pine nuts, etc.)
>> ¼ cup freshly grated Parmesan, Pecorino, or Romano cheese (optional)
>> Freshly ground black pepper and salt or dulse flakes

To make the pesto:
Combine the herbs, garlic, and olive oil in a blender or food processor and pulse until creamy. Mix in the sunflower seeds, cheese (if using), and salt and pepper to taste.

To use:
Serve on toast or crackers, pasta, steamed grains, omelets, or vegetables.

Thyme / *Thymus vulgaris*

Oddly, this diminutive, fragrant herb is beloved by gardeners and bees alike and has a long and respected medicinal past but is neglected by many contemporary herbalists. I think it's one of our best medicines. It's one of my favorite cold and cough remedies; I've often used it to make a delicious and effective cough syrup. Dr. Paul Lee, a professor at the University of California at Santa Cruz, did a number of studies on thyme and found that it has a major strengthening effect on the thymus gland, thereby enhancing immune function. Lee became widely known for his thyme salve and his famous "thymus thump":

he'd apply generous amounts of his homemade salve over his thymus gland and then, Tarzan fashion, thump his upper chest, where the thymus gland is located. As bizarre as this may sound, the "thymus thump" has been proved to stimulate thymus gland activity, perhaps much in the same way that knowledgeable gardeners know to stimulate plant growth by shaking their pots or brushing the tops of their plants to simulate stress.

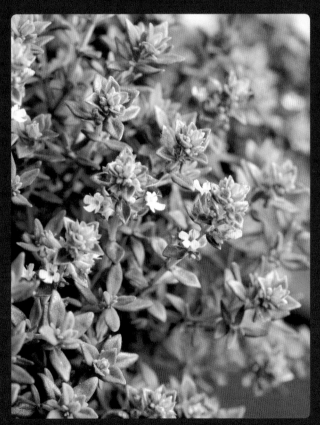

GROWING THYME

Thyme is a hardy perennial that seems to thrive in most climates, though it prefers well-drained, alkaline soil and a sunny location. Seeds can be sown directly in the soil in the late spring or indoors in flats for an earlier start. There are many varieties of thyme, some which grow upright and others that are creepers. For medicinal purposes, choose common garden thyme (*Thymus vulgaris*) and/or lemon thyme (*T. citriodorus*), my favorite thyme for tea. As the plant matures, it becomes woody and benefits from heavy trimming in the early spring, before new growth commences. Trimming will keep your thyme happy. Just talking about more thyme makes me happy.

MEDICINAL USES

Thyme is a powerful and effective disinfectant and can be used both externally (as a wash) and internally to help fight off infection. It's often used to help ward off colds and as a rinse to treat sore throat and oral infections. It also makes a fine tea for treating coughs and chest complaints and is used in many antifungal remedies. A recent study shows that it's rich in antioxidants (most plants are) and has a markedly tonic effect, supporting normal body functions. It seems to have a positive effect on the glandular system as a whole, and especially the thymus gland.

Parts used
Leaf and flower

Key constituents
Essential oil with variable constituents (thymol, cineole, borneol), flavonoids, tannins

Safety factor
Thyme is completely safe and nontoxic.

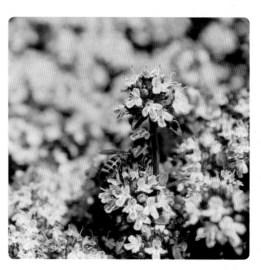

Trimming thyme plants in early spring will encourage more flowers, making the bees happy, too!

Thyme Syrup

This is one of my favorite syrups for treating coughs, colds, and chest complaints. I bought my first bottle of thyme syrup in a small market in the south of France, and I've been hooked ever since. It's very effective medicine, but also delicious enough to add to sparkling water and serve as a sparkling thyme tisane.

» 2-4 ounces thyme leaf and flower (fresh is best but dried will do)

» 1 quart water

» 1 cup honey

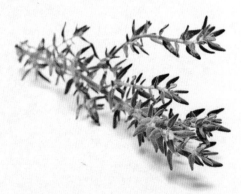

To make the syrup:
Combine the thyme and water in a pan over very low heat. Simmer lightly, with the lid ajar to allow the steam to escape, until the liquid is reduced by half, giving you about 2 cups of strong thyme tea. Strain, and compost the spent herbs. Add the honey to the warm liquid and stir, just until the honey is melted. Store in a glass jar in the refrigerator, where the honey will keep for 3 to 4 weeks.

To use:
Take ½ to 1 teaspoon every couple of hours until the cold or cough subsides.

. . . .

Variation

For a longer shelf life, add ¼ cup of brandy to each cup of syrup. Brandy not only is a good preservative but also serves as an antispasmodic and will help relax the throat muscles, which is helpful in treating a cough.

Thyme Honey

Thyme honey probably wouldn't be considered the strongest remedy for coughs and colds, but it is one of the better tasting.

To make the honey:

Fill a widemouthed glass jar half full of fresh thyme leaves and flowers. Gently warm a batch of raw, unpasteurized honey, so that it will better extract the properties of the thyme. Do not overheat or boil; heat over 110°F will kill the honey's enzymes and destroy its medicinal benefit. Add enough honey to the jar to cover the herbs, and place the jar in a warm spot (near a sunny window will work). Let steep for approximately 2 weeks. (You could also use a slow cooker set to 100°F. It will take only a few hours of constant warm heat to make a strong medicinal honey.)

When the honey tastes and smells strongly of thyme, it's finished. You can leave the tiny thyme leaves in the honey, which is what I do. Of course you can also strain them out for a more professional look, but it can be messy! Bottle and store in a cool pantry or in the refrigerator, where the honey will keep for several months.

To use:

Use by the teaspoonful. Enjoy this delicious thyme honey by itself, or use it to sweeten teas for additional medicinal benefits.

Variation

For additional flavor, add 4 to 6 drops of pure essential lemon oil to each cup of thyme honey. Delicious!

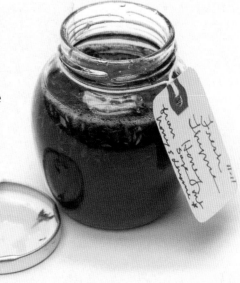

A close cousin to ginger, turmeric is native to India and South Asia, and its bright yellow color and pungent flavor are well-recognized features of classic Indian and Asian dishes. Although it is a highly regarded medicine in its native regions, its powerful healing properties have been largely ignored by the rest of the world until recently. Which is too bad, because turmeric is among the most antioxidant-rich, anti-inflammatory, and immune-enhancing herbs available.

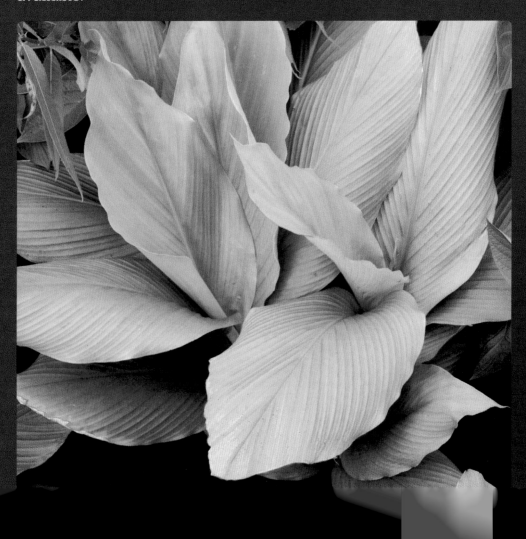

GROWING TURMERIC

Turmeric thrives in warm, moist, tropical conditions. It can be grown in a pot, but be sure the pot is large, as it can grow 3 to 5 feet tall. Plant the rhizome shallowly in rich soil, and keep moist, warm, and in full sunshine. Turmeric has stunning bright red flowers that are gorgeous in a garden setting.

MEDICINAL USES

Traditionally, turmeric was used in both Ayurvedic and traditional Chinese medicine as a remedy for jaundice and other liver and gallbladder disorders. As a pungent, dry, warming herb, it was also used to treat chest colds and coughs. It was also highly valued for its powerful anti-inflammatory properties, which modern research has shown to work by sensitizing the body's cortisol receptor sites, making turmeric an effective treatment for arthritis, osteoarthritis, and most other inflammatory conditions. According to recent studies, it is stronger acting than hydrocortisone, without any of the harmful side effects.

Curcumin, one of turmeric's major constituents, is an effective topical antibacterial agent and has stronger antioxidant properties than vitamin E. Curcumin is also proving to be a powerful agent against several types of cancer, including breast, colon, prostate, and skin cancers. In 2009 the *British Journal of Cancer* published a study showing that curcumin was effective in killing esophageal cancer cells within 24 hours of treatment. Other recent study has shown promising results in turmeric's ability to inhibit growth of lymphoma cells.

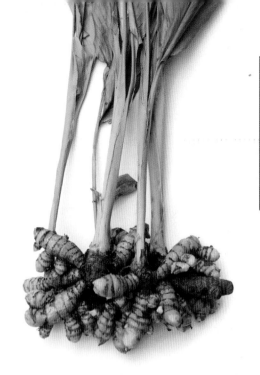

A close cousin to ginger, turmeric has many of the same uses, but it is also immune enhancing and a powerful anti-inflammatory.

Part used

Rhizome

Key constituents

Essential oils (containing zingiberene and turmerone), curcumin, bitters, resins

Safety factor

None; it's been a popular spice for centuries. However, turmeric is very warming and drying. If you find its properties to be too drying or warming, try combining it with a moisture-enhancing herb, such as marsh mallow root, or increase your water intake.

And clinical trials conducted in China in the late 1980s indicate that turmeric helps lower blood cholesterol and has anti-coagulant action that can help prevent the formation of harmful blood clots that could lead to stroke.

One of turmeric's most common uses is as a digestive aid. A warming, pungent, somewhat bitter herb, it stimulates the flow of bile, which aids in the digestion of fats and oils. It also helps stabilize the digestive system's microflora, thus inhibiting yeast overgrowth. No wonder it's popular in so many dishes around the world.

Hailed in many parts of the world as an effective immune-enhancing herb, turmeric has in the past been overlooked in North America, perhaps because of the huge popularity and renown of echinacea. But its reputation for supporting the immune system has been upheld for centuries, and as it becomes more widely propagated and readily available, it's becoming more popular in the United States as an herb to benefit immune-system function.

Golden Milk

This is a traditional Ayurvedic healing drink used to treat inflammation, such as in arthritis and bursitis, and to support the immune system.

» ¼ cup turmeric root powder

» Almond oil

» Milk (cow's, almond, or coconut)

» Honey (optional)

To make the turmeric base:
Combine the turmeric with ½ cup water in a saucepan. Bring to a boil, then lower the heat and simmer until the mixture turns into a thick paste. Cool, scoop into a glass jar, and store in the refrigerator.

To use:
To make one serving, combine ½ to 1 teaspoon turmeric paste, 1 teaspoon almond oil, and 1 cup milk in a blender. Add honey to sweeten, if you wish. Blend to make a frothy drink.

Variation

You can add other herbs to this basic recipe, simmering them with the turmeric. Traditional additions include adaptogenic tonics, such as ashwagandha, astragalus, cinnamon, and ginger.

Golden Turmeric Paste for Skin Infections

This paste is an effective treatment for a variety of skin infections, including fungal infections such as athlete's foot and ringworm. It's interesting to note that many of the herbs that are effective against fungal infections are also very colorful and stain the skin. Is there some special antibacterial/antifungal action in the pigments? In any case, this turmeric paste will work, but be prepared for brightly colored skin. The stain will last for a few days and then slowly fade.

» 1 tablespoon goldenseal root powder (organically cultivated)

» 1 tablespoon turmeric root powder

» Rubbing alcohol or turmeric tincture

» 6–8 drops tea tree and/or eucalyptus essential oil

To make the paste:
Combine the herbs with enough rubbing alcohol to form a paste. Add the essential oil. Store in an airtight container; the paste will keep for several weeks.

To use:
Apply directly to the infected skin once or twice a day until the infection is gone. Ringworm, athlete's foot, and other minor infections will respond within a week or two, but tenacious fungal infections such as nail infections can require a much longer treatment and other herbal remedies as well.

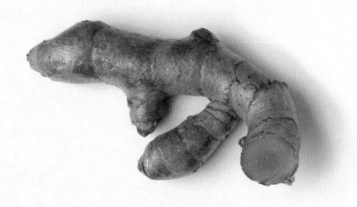

Medicinal Curry Blend

I love when medicine and food are one and the same. And so it is with curry powder. Every herb used in a traditional curry is a well-known medicinal plant. Often these herbs became part of the recipe as much for their medicinal properties as for their flavor. Curry powder contains warming, drying, anti-bacterial herbs that aid digestion, fight bacterial infections, and help stabilize blood sugar levels while increasing microflora activity. Because it's warming and drying, curry is also useful for treating colds and chest complaints. This recipe is shared by Kathi Keville, author of The Illustrated Herb Encyclopedia.

» 1 ounce coriander seed

» 1 ounce cumin seed

» 1 ounce turmeric root

» ½ ounce black mustard seed

» ½ ounce chile pepper

» ½ ounce fennel seed

» ½ ounce ginger root

Note: *Spices are always best freshly ground from whole dried herbs. For convenience and ease, you can use powdered herbs for this mix, but truly, a really fine mix is made by grinding the herbs as you need them.*

To make the curry blend:
If any of the herbs are in whole form, grind them to a powder. Combine the spices with a small amount of oil (¼ cup of oil for every 2 to 3 teaspoons of herbs) in a saucepan and warm over very low heat for a few minutes, until the herbs are fragrant. You can use the spice blend as is, or you can add enough coconut milk or water to make a paste. Store in the refrigerator, where the blend will keep for several weeks.

To use:
To treat a cold or respiratory problem, add 1 teaspoon to cup of miso soup. To treat sluggish digestion and bowels, add 1 tablespoon to food as needed. Curry is great served on rice or vegetables or mixed with oil and vinegar as a dressing. And, of course, you can use this blend in any traditional curry dish.

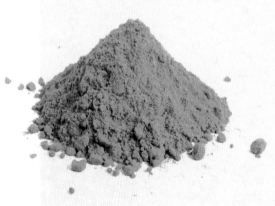

OTHER USEFUL KITCHEN HERBS & SPICES

The common kitchen herbs and spices presented here are not necessarily less important than the ones described in more detail earlier, but they are, perhaps, not as diverse or used as often.

ARUGULA. Considered a sexual stimulant and reproductive tonic, arugula is nutrient dense, containing high levels of iron, calcium, magnesium, and trace minerals. It has a sophisticated hot, almost bitter flavor that might take some getting used to, but this is a green worth knowing.

BLACK PEPPER. One of the great tonics in traditional Chinese medicine, black pepper is warming, energizing, and stimulating. It is indicated for "cold-type" problems such as flus, coughs, colds, poor circulation, and poor digestion.

CARDAMOM. With a divinely sensual flavor, cardamom belongs to the same esteemed family as ginger and turmeric. It stimulates the mind and arouses the senses. In Ayurvedic medicine, it is considered one of the safest and best digestive aids.

CLOVE. Clove has long been used to relieve the pain of toothache and oral infection. Its essential oil contains high levels of acetyleugenol, a powerful antiseptic and antispasmodic. Clove also has antifungal properties and is often used in antifungal remedies.

DILL. An effective and well-known remedy for digestive complaints, gas, and hiccups, dill has powerful antispasmodic properties. At one time it was the most well-known herb for soothing colicky babies.

HORSERADISH. My number-one favorite remedy for sinus congestion and head colds. Nothing works better! The root is rich in minerals, including silica, as well as vitamins, including vitamin C. Its warming antiseptic properties make it the herb of choice for treating asthma, catarrh, lung infections, and other congestive conditions.

MARJORAM/OREGANO. Both marjoram and oregano are used to relieve nervousness, irritability, and insomnia due to tension and anxiety. They are both powerful antiseptic and disinfectant herbs that effectively fight bacterial and viral infections.

MINT. Most mints are rich in essential oils, vitamin C, beta-carotene, and chlorophyll. They are generally excellent antispasmodics and are useful for preventing cramps and muscle spasms.

PARSLEY. Rich in iron, beta-carotene, chlorophyll, and many other vitamins and minerals, parsley is used to treat iron deficiency, anemia, and fatigue. A primary herb for bladder and kidney problems, it is a safe and effective diuretic. It can help to dry up a mother's milk during the weaning process and is effective as a poultice for swollen, enlarged breasts and/or mastitis. (Of course, if a nursing mother does not want to decrease her milk supply, she should not consume parsley in great quantities.)

CHAPTER 4

24 Safe & Effective Herbs to Know, Grow, and Use

Have you ever walked into an herb shop or the herb section of a natural foods store and marveled at all those jars of colorful herbs? Wondered what they were used for? Where they came from? There is something about herbal medicine that is enticing, even mysterious and magical, and we often find ourselves wanting to know more . . . but where do we begin?

There's no better way to learn about herbal medicine than to create your own small apothecary, be it a pantry shelf, a closet, an extra room, or a corner of the basement, and fill it with homemade herbal remedies, ideally prepared from plants you've grown yourself so you can observe them through the seasons. Now you're ready to begin practicing family herbalism. If you think this sounds daunting, remember, it's called *practice* because that's exactly what you'll be doing: practicing how to use herbs to promote vibrant health and radiant well-being.

All of the medicinal plants described in this chapter, while effective and active, are safe and nontoxic, with few if any negative side effects, so you can use them with confidence, getting to know them as you work with them. And most of these herbs, as you'll discover, will grow well whether you're living in the big city and gardening in pots or "at home on the range" in the desert. These plants are survivors, and with just a little care they'll thrive. So, let's get started.

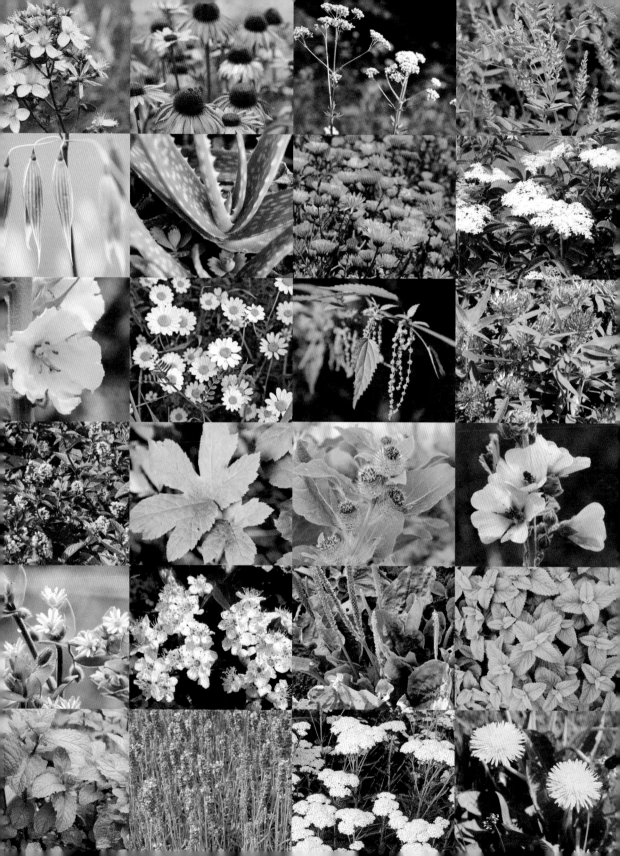

Aloe Vera / *Aloe barbadensis*

This handsome East African native has wound its way around the globe and is now as popular — and happy, it seems — in garden designs as it is potbound on the kitchen windowsill. It has become so popular, in fact, that you can find this juicy green succulent for sale even in supermarkets and big box stores. But, I wonder, how many people have taken advantage of the healing wonders of this plant?

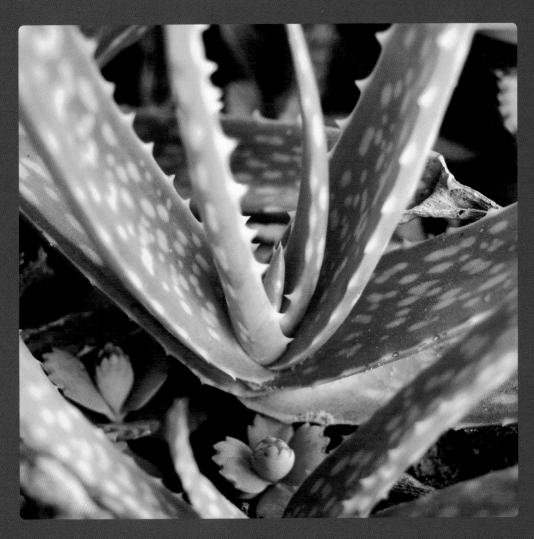

GROWING ALOE VERA

An aloe plant is a must in every household. Its large, succulent, bladelike leaves make it a handsome potted plant; sitting in a sunny south-facing window, it will grow for many seasons with little care. Though aloe is a sun-loving native of the warm, dry regions of the world, it is quite hardy and can survive outdoors in Zone 8 if well protected. Aloe prefers full sun, sandy and well-drained soil, and moderate watering, but it is quite tolerant and will grow in a variety of less-than-ideal conditions. I have been known to move pots of aloe out of the house in the late spring to a shady part of the garden (to avoid having them "sunburned") and then shamefully forget about them. Months later, when I rediscover them, neglected in the full shade, overwatered by the endless summer rains, they are still alive, albeit in need of a little TLC.

Aloe is simply one of the easiest houseplants to grow. My friend and fellow herbalist Brigitte Mars writes, "If you can't grow aloe, then try plastic plants." A bit harsh, but I would agree, it's almost that easy. Give it sunshine, well-drained soil, and only moderate water, and your aloe should thrive, rewarding you with an endless abundance of healing leaves.

MEDICINAL USES

Aloe is truly a remarkable healing agent for burns, both superficial (first degree) and serious (second and third degree). Applied topically, the thick gel that oozes from the cut leaves is soothing and pain relieving, and it contains rich concentrations of anthraquinones, which promote rapid healing and tissue repair. A thick application of aloe vera gel not only soothes and cools a kitchen burn or really bad sunburn but also quickly reverses the blisters and prevents scarring and tissue damage. It is also helpful in cases of insect bites and stings, rashes, eczema, acne, skin ulcers, and the inflammation caused by poison oak and poison ivy.

Aloe is said to have been a favorite herb of Cleopatra. Perhaps the world's first "beauty queen" and cosmetics entrepreneur, Cleopatra popularized many famous beauty products, including milk and oats for bathing and aloe for skin care. Did Cleopatra know that aloe gel contains a natural sunscreen that blocks 20 to 30 percent of ultraviolet rays, or that it perfectly matches the natural pH of our skin, making it a near-perfect skin tonic? Rumor has it that aloe was the "secret ingredient" in Cleopatra's face cream. It's certainly a not-so-secret ingredient in Rosemary's Famous Face Cream (see page 116).

Taken internally, aloe vera is one of the most widely used and safe laxatives. The laxative action derives from the aloin, or bitter constituents, found in the outer sheath of the leaf blades. The aloin is often dried, powdered, and added to commercial laxatives. You should be careful when using aloe as a laxative, though, as it is quite powerful and can have purgative effects, causing intestinal cramping and pain if used in excess.

The juice or gel of the pulp within the leaves is one of the most healing, soothing remedies for digestive irritation and inflammation, such as stomach ulcers and colitis. It's also a well-known remedy for arthritic pain and bursitis, whether taken internally or applied externally as a liniment. It effectively cools heat and soothes inflammation, not only easing the pain but also actually helping to heal the underlying cause.

For internal use, you can scoop aloe gel directly from fresh aloe leaves, but be certain to avoid the skin and outermost layer of the leaves, to avoid the laxative properties. Though I have many potted aloe plants and use the leaves freely for skin irritations, burns, and wounds, I keep a jar of commercially prepared aloe vera gel in the refrigerator for internal purposes. It's handy for soothing intestinal problems, arthritic pain,

and inflammation, without the worry about the laxative properties. Aloe is rather bland tasting, perhaps a bit on the bitter side, but it can be nicely flavored with a bit of lemon juice or added to a cup of fruit or vegetable juice; you hardly notice the flavor.

Commercial aloe vera gel is also the best choice for creams and lotions, since fresh aloe gel will spoil rather quickly. Commercial aloe generally has ascorbic acid added as a natural preservative, which will give your creams and lotions a longer shelf life.

Parts used

Leaves and pressed juice (or gel)

Key constituents

Fiber, B vitamins, vitamin E, selenium, silicon, enzymes, aloin, anthraquinones, polysaccharides, tannins

Safety factors

The dried powder and outer leaf sheath of aloe can be very strong laxatives and purgatives; always follow dosage instructions when using it for laxative purposes. Because of its strong laxative properties, pregnant or nursing mothers should avoid using aloe internally, and it should be given to the elderly and children with caution. If cramping or stomach pain occurs, discontinue use.

Aloe is not recommended as a topical treatment for staph or staph-related infections such as impetigo. It seals in the staph bacteria, creating a perfect petri dish for them to grow in. If you suspect staph, don't use an aloe-based cream or ointment.

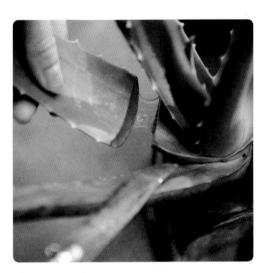

The inner gel of the aloe leaf is wonderfully soothing and an effective healing remedy for wounds.

Aloe Vera Gel

For soothing burns, wounds, and skin irritations, nothing beats fresh aloe vera gel.

To prepare the gel:

Cut a large, firm leaf from your aloe plant. Slice it open; it's best to do this on a plate, because as soon as you slice into aloe, it will begin to ooze its gel. Use a tablespoon to scoop out the inner gel. If you want a smooth gel (optional), purée it in a blender. Store the gel in a small bottle in the refrigerator, where it will keep for at least several weeks. (According to *The Illustrated Herb Encyclopedia*, by Kathi Keville, to further extend aloe gel's shelf life, add 500 IU of vitamin C per cup of gel.)

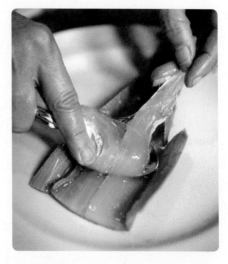

To use:

Apply the gel directly to a burn, wound, or skin irritation. It will feel cooling and soothing and will begin immediately to repair and heal damaged tissue. As the aloe dries, it will begin to pull and tighten the skin. This is part of the healing process, but if it becomes uncomfortable, gently rinse the aloe off. Repeat the application several times a day.

Variations

* You can also leave the gel in the leaf, cutting off only as much as you need for each application. Wrap the leaf in waxed paper or plastic wrap to keep it fresh and to keep the gel from oozing out. Stored this way, the aloe leaf will remain fresh and active for several days or even weeks.

* Make an aloe-spearmint juice for healing and soothing by combining 1 cup aloe vera gel (from inner leaf; do not use outer leaf) with juice from 1 lemon and a few fresh spearmint sprigs. Place in a blender and blend thoroughly. Sweeten with a spoonful of honey if you want to, but I rather enjoy the tart, refreshing flavor. Drink ¼ to ½ cup as needed throughout the day. (For added zest and digestive enzymes, mix in ½ cup unsweetened pineapple juice.)

Healing Aloe Lotion for Poison Oak & Poison Ivy

You can use commercially prepared aloe or homemade gel (see recipe on page 105). For homemade gel, be sure to preserve it with 500 IU of vitamin C per cup. As a complementary therapy to help relieve the stress and pain caused by poison oak and ivy, take 1 teaspoon of valerian tincture as needed throughout the day.

» 1 part burdock leaf
» 1 part plantain leaf
» 1 part yarrow leaf and flower
» Apple cider vinegar (preferably unpasteurized)
» Aloe vera gel
» Peppermint essential oil

To make the lotion:
Fill a glass pint jar with equal parts burdock, plantain, and yarrow and then fill the jar with apple cider vinegar. Let sit in a warm, sunny window for 2 to 3 weeks. Strain, reserving the liquid. For each cup of herbal vinegar, add ½ cup aloe vera gel and 4 or 5 drops of peppermint essential oil.

To use:
Shake well before using. Apply topically to soothe, cool, and heal the rash and itchiness.

Aloe-Comfrey Arthritis Gel

» comfrey root and leaf
» ¼ cup aloe vera gel
» 1–2 drops spearmint, peppermint, or wintergreen essential oil

To make the gel:
Make ¼ cup of strong comfrey tea as an infusion, following the instructions on page 29. Combine with the aloe vera gel and essential oil, mixing well. Store in a glass jar in the refrigerator, where it will keep for 5 to 7 days.

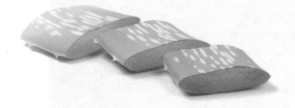

To use:
Shake well before using. Apply topically to sore muscles and arthritic joints, massaging it in gently.

This tenacious wild plant is a bane to farmers but a blessing to herbalists. It is quite simply one of the safest, tastiest, and most effective detoxifying and cleansing herbs in Western and traditional Chinese medicine. Best of all, it grows in a wide range of conditions and habitats and is free for the picking!

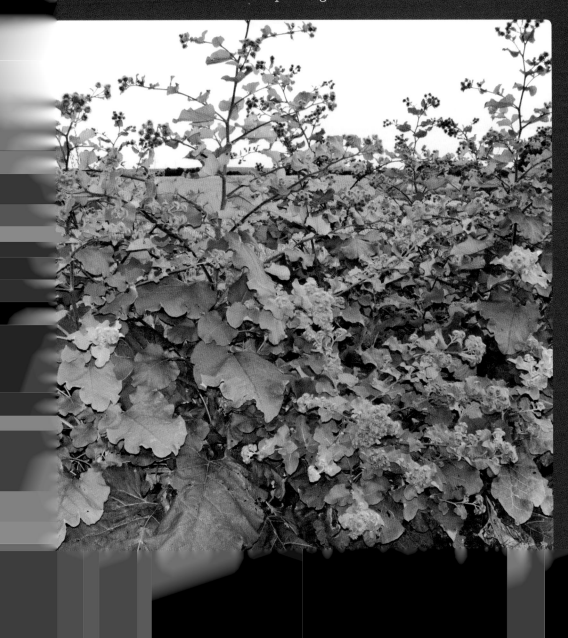

GROWING BURDOCK

For most people, the question is how *not* to grow burdock. It is a happily aggressive, tenacious weed that thrives across the continent. Its round, prickly seedpod, cleverly designed to attach to whatever passes by — animal, bird, person, it's not fussy — is a highly effective mechanism of seed dispersal, and was the inspiration behind Velcro. Burdock is an easy grower and will do well in poor soil, fertile soil, rocky soil, or what have you. It survives freezing temperatures but does equally well in warmer weather. It is drought resistant but appreciates a bit of rain now and again. A large, vigorous plant, with huge broad leaves and thistlelike flowers, it's quite handsome in the garden. However, burdock produces hundreds of seeds in those pods, so if you don't want a garden full of burdock, clip the seeds in the fall before they ripen. And if you have pets, especially pets with long hair, you'll definitely want to clip those burdock seeds or expect to shave your pet. I've watered socks that were hopelessly embedded with burdock and had them sprout!

MEDICINAL USES

Burdock is one of the best herbs for skin problems and can be used internally and externally to treat eczema, psoriasis, and other skin-related imbalances. It is my favorite herb for teenagers who have problem skin, acne, boils, and other "hot conditions" due to the shifting hormones of the teen years, and sometimes due to too rich a diet (too much sugar and fast food). Burdock may not be the only remedy needed to

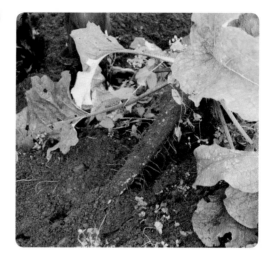

The burdock root is a versatile and powerful healing agent.

fully correct the problem, but it will noticeably help — if you can convince your teenager to try it. It helps that burdock is rather pleasant tasting. Get your teenager to try Root Beer Tea, mixed with sparkling water (see page 110); it's flavored with ginger, cinnamon, and stevia (for sweetness) and tastes like an old-fashioned root beer. Or give your teen a burdock tincture, if that's easier. The best remedy in the world does no good if it sits on the shelf.

Burdock also makes an effective wash for dry, itchy, irritated skin. Decoct the root, and apply a cloth soaked in the tea directly to the skin. Or use the tea in the bathwater.

Burdock is a specific remedy for the liver, and it's also "cooling," which is useful for hot, agitated conditions. Got a husband who gets angry, is often hot and red, and has signs of "liver stress" — poor digestion, gas, perhaps a little overweight? Then burdock would be the herb of choice. Make a

Parts used

Primarily the root, though the seeds and leaves are used externally as poultices and salves

Key constituents

Calcium, magnesium, phosphorus, iron and chromium, inulin, sesquiterpenes, bitter glycosides, flavonoids, volatile oils

Safety factor

None; burdock is among the safest and most widely used herbs.

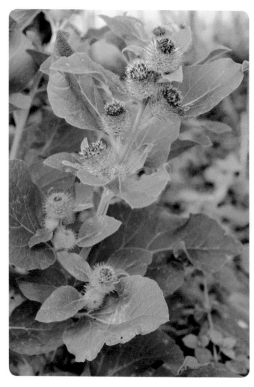

The burdock seeds are used in salves and poultices for soothing skin rashes.

tincture using equal parts burdock root and dandelion root. Have him take 1 teaspoon two or three times a day for 4 to 6 weeks. Of course, it would help if he would also cut back on fried foods, red meat, and cheese, but even just the burdock-and-dandelion mix can be helpful for nourishing and toning the liver and reducing symptoms of "heat" (signified by red face, hot temper, and hot, flushed skin).

Scientists are studying burdock root's anticancer, antitumor potential. The root is part of a very well-known Native American anticancer formula called Essiac, a formula still available and used today. And burdock root is known to have a beneficial effect on the lymphatic system, which is an important part of the immune system. Burdock is recommended whenever there is lymph stagnation or congestion, indicated by swollen lymph nodes throughout the body. Have swollen lymph glands?

Drink 3 to 4 cups of burdock tea a day for it to effectively cleanse your system. That seems like a lot of tea, doesn't it? It is, but it helps cut back on other drinks that are not so healthy. Make a quart of tea a day and carry it with you. By day's end, it should be gone. And after 1 or 2 days, the swollen lymph glands should be gone as well.

Root Beer Tea

This recipe can be made with fresh or dried roots. It's sweetened with stevia, a small shrub whose green leaves are exceedingly sweet — 50 times sweeter than sugar. Stevia has no calories and causes no harm to teeth or gums, and causes no harm to diabetics and others with blood sugar issues. It's used in many parts of the world as a healthy alternative to sugar. Why don't we see it more in this country? The sugar industry is a huge lobbying force in Washington.

- 1 part burdock root, chopped
- 1 part cinnamon chips
- 1 part sarsaparilla root
- ½ part dandelion root (the more the better, but it will make the tea a little bitter)
- ¼ part gingerroot, chopped (not powdered) or freshly grated
- A pinch of stevia (½ teaspoon per quart is generally sufficient)
- Sparkling water (optional)

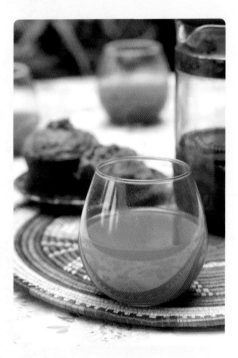

To make the tea:
Prepare a decoction of the burdock, cinnamon, sarsaparilla, dandelion, and ginger, following the instructions on page 30 and adjusting the flavors as suits your own taste. Strain. Drink warm or cool. It's delicious when mixed with sparkling water — ¼ cup of sparking water to ¾ cup of tea, poured over ice.

To use:
This tea is good enough to drink for pleasure, but for medicinal purposes, such as treating acne or eczema, drink 2 to 3 cups daily for 2 weeks, stop for a week, and repeat as needed.

Steamed Gobo (Burdock Root)

This popular dish can be found in fine Japanese restaurants.

To prepare the dish:
Clean fresh burdock roots, and peel if the outside seems particularly tough. Grate the root. Steam lightly (for just 3 to 5 minutes), sprinkle with toasted sesame seed oil, and stir well. Garnish with toasted sesame seeds, if desired.

To use:
Eat! This is "medicine" at its finest.

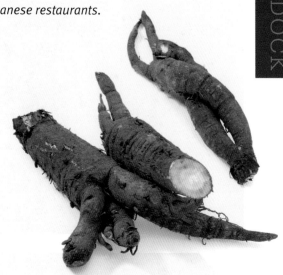

Cooling Liver Tincture

Too much heat in the system? An overly hot condition is indicated by a red or ruddy complexion, agitation, hot temper, and an often "fired-up" personality. Heat is good in the body, but too much heat can cause hypertension, heart problems, and liver disorders.

» 1 part burdock root
» 1 part dandelion root
» ¼ part cinnamon bark
» 80-proof alcohol, unpasteurized apple cider vinegar, or glycerin

To make the tincture:
Prepare a tincture with the herbs, following the instructions on page 40.

To use:
Take ½ to 1 teaspoon three or four times a day for 4 to 6 weeks. You can continue taking the tincture for longer, if necessary. Burdock, dandelion, and cinnamon are considered "medicinal foods" with no harmful side effects, even over the long term.

Calendula / *Calendula officinalis*

This sunny little flower brightens many a garden. Not only hardy and beautiful, the radiant yellow flowers are amazingly healing. They're also edible. Calendula flowers were at one time a frequent ingredient in winter stews and soups; because the plants have an extended blooming season (year-round, in some warmer locales), the flowers were thought to promote a sunny disposition and good health through the colder months. If calendula is blooming in your garden, don't serve a salad without adorning it with calendula's golden rays. They will brighten any meal and make even the most reluctant of salad eaters head back for seconds. Try an omelet with steamed nettle, feta, and calendula blossoms for a gourmet treat.

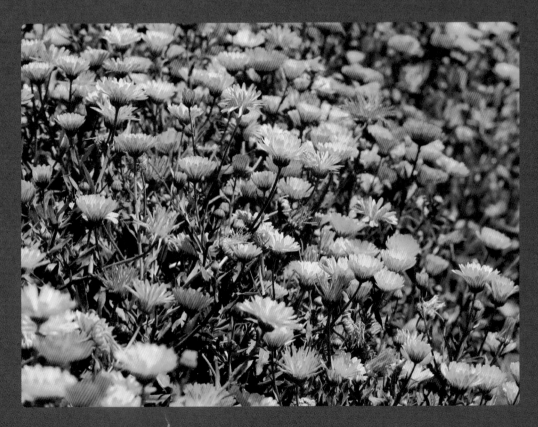

GROWING CALENDULA

Calendula may be the most rewarding flower you grow. It starts blooming early and is often still bravely blooming as the first snows fall in our northern Vermont garden. Sow seeds directly in the garden. In more temperate climates you can sow in the fall for an early-spring bloom. In Vermont, though some of my calendula does self-sow and return in the spring, I usually collect seeds in the fall and plant them in the spring. The more you pick those bright orbs of gold and yellow, the more the plant blooms. Unlike many flowers, this gorgeous girl is not fussy. It likes full sunshine, good fertile soil (though it will do okay in poor soil as well), and occasional watering. It will do well if pampered, and almost as well if ignored. When the blossoms are ready to pick, they are sticky with resin (the resin has many antifungal properties, so sticky flowers are good).

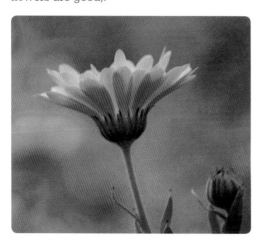

Calendula is one of the hardiest flowers in the garden, often continuing to bloom even after the first snowfall.

MEDICINAL USES

Calendula flower is a powerful vulnerary, healing wounds by promoting cell repair and growth. The flower is also a noted antiseptic and anti-inflammatory. Applied topically or used internally, it can help keep infections at bay, and it's a common ingredient in creams, salves, and ointments for treating bruises, burns, sores, skin ulcers, skin infections, and rashes. Calendula flower is a wonderful herb for babies, being potent as well as soothing and gentle. It is one of the most popular herbs for treating cradle cap, diaper rash, and other skin irritations. And calendula tea is a useful remedy for thrush, a type of yeast overgrowth not uncommon in infants.

Calendula tea is also useful both internally and externally (as a wash or poultice) to moderate fever, keeping it from rising too high. The flower's mild astringent and antiseptic properties are helpful for treating gastrointestinal problems such as ulcers (mixed with marsh mallow root) and cramps (mixed with valerian or cramp bark), indigestion (mixed with peppermint), and diarrhea (alone or mixed with blackberry root).

Calendula is one of the best herbs for nourishing and cleansing the lymphatic system. This is the first herb I turn to for treating swollen glands. Alone or mixed with other lymph cleansers such as burdock, red clover, cleavers, and chickweed, calendula works to stimulate lymphatic drainage and move congestion out of the body. The lymph system is an important part of the immune system, but it has no pumping mechanism and so depends on movement of the body to encourage the lymph fluid to move easily and quickly. Are you stretching, dancing, jumping, exercising? If not, the lymph nodes can easily become congested and sluggish. Drink calendula, red clover, and burdock tea and get moving for healthy-flowing lymph!

Part used

Flower

Key constituents

Carotenoids, flavonoids, mucilage, saponins, bitters, volatile oil, resins

Safety factor

Calendula has a perfect safety record, with no toxity reported. Use with joy and ease.

Calendula Oil

Pick the calendula buds when they are just opening, if possible on a dry and sunny day, when the resin will be stronger. Your fingers may become sticky from the resin while you're picking the buds. That's a good sign.

To make the oil:

Fill a glass quart jar three-quarters full with calendula buds. Fill the jar to within an inch of the top with olive oil (for medicinal preparations) or grapeseed, almond, or apricot kernel oil (for cosmetic preparations). Place in a warm, sunny spot, and let the herbs and oil infuse for 3 to 4 weeks. Strain and rebottle. (For double-strength calendula oil, add a fresh batch of calendula buds to the strained oil and let infuse for another 3 to 4 weeks.) Store in a cool place, out of direct sunlight (the refrigerator is fine), where the oil will keep for up to a year.

To use:

Apply calendula oil topically to skin rashes, eczema, and swollen lymph glands. It makes a wonderful massage oil and is a great addition to any cosmetic recipe calling for oil.

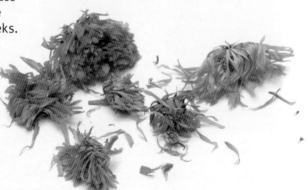

Calendula Salve

This is a favorite salve of most herbalists and is used for treating all manner of skin problems, such as wounds, cuts, and rashes. It is also a great salve for treating cradle cap and diaper rash in infants and toddlers. The lavender essential oil adds not just scent but also antibacterial, antifungal, and antimicrobial properties.

» 1 cup Calendula Oil (see recipe, page 114)

» ¼ cup grated beeswax

» 4–6 drops lavender essential oil

» 1 pinch of turmeric root powder (for color)

To make the salve:
Warm the oil over very low heat and stir in most of the beeswax, reserving just a tablespoon. As soon as the beeswax has melted, put a tablespoon of the mix on a plate in the freezer for a minute or two, until the salve cools. Check the consistency. If you decide you want a firmer salve, add the rest of the beeswax. If you want a softer salve, add a little more oil.

When the salve has reached your preferred consistency, add the essential oil, using more or less depending on the strength of scent you prefer. Stir in turmeric to enhance the orange color.

Pour into small jars or tins. Let cool, then put the lids on the jars and store in a cool, dark location, where the salve will keep for at least a year.

To use:
Apply a small amount of calendula salve topically to treat skin rashes, wounds, cuts, diaper rash, or cradle cap, massaging it gently into the affected area.

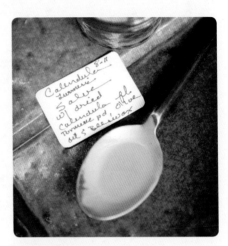

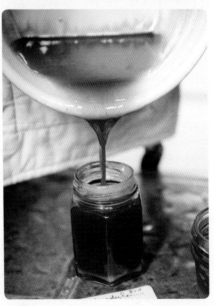

Rosemary's Famous Face Cream

This rich, thick cream is wonderfully moisturizing, and it is probably one of my most famous formulas. It's the perfect face cream, and depending on the herbs added, it can be very healing for skin problems. Made with calendula oil and essential oil of lavender, for example, it can be used as a healing cream for babies, as a soothing remedy for rough or irritated skin, or simply as a divine cosmetic for mature and "sageing" skin.

>> ¾ cup Calendula Oil, made with equal parts grapeseed and apricot kernel oil (see recipe, page 114)

>> ⅛ cup cocoa butter

>> ⅛ cup coconut oil

>> 1 rounded tablespoon grated beeswax

>> ¼ cup commercially prepared aloe vera gel

>> ¾ cup distilled water

>> A few drops of lavender essential oil

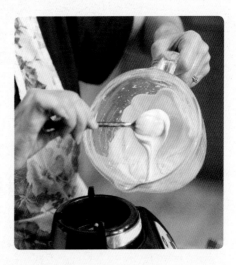

To make the cream:

Combine the calendula oil, cocoa butter, coconut oil, and beeswax in a saucepan over very low heat and warm until everything is melted together. Pour into a measuring cup or bowl and let cool for at least several hours or overnight, until the mixture is somewhat firm, thick, and creamy.

Scrape oil mixture into a blender. In a separate bowl, combine the aloe vera gel, distilled water, and essential oil. Turn the blender on at high speed and slowly drizzle the water mixture into the oil, continuing to blend until all the water mixture has been absorbed by the oil. The blender should "choke" as the mixture thickens and becomes white and creamy.

Turn off the blender and scoop the cream into small jars. Apply the lids and store in a cool, dark location, where the cream will keep for up to a year.

To use:

Apply this rich, thick cream as often as you like. Because it's quite inexpensve to make, you can use your "face cream" for your whole body! It does wonders for dry and sensitive skin.

Chamomile / *Chamaemelum nobile, Matricaria recutita, and related species*

This well-known and highly respected plant is a healing wonder. Chamomile demonstrates to us that gentle does not mean less effective; though exceedingly gentle, it is also potent and effective. The pharmacopoeias (official medical documents or authorities) of 26 countries have approved chamomile to treat conditions ranging from colic and indigestion to muscle spasms, tension, inflammation, and infection. Though small in stature, chamomile looms large in any home herbalist's medicine cabinet.

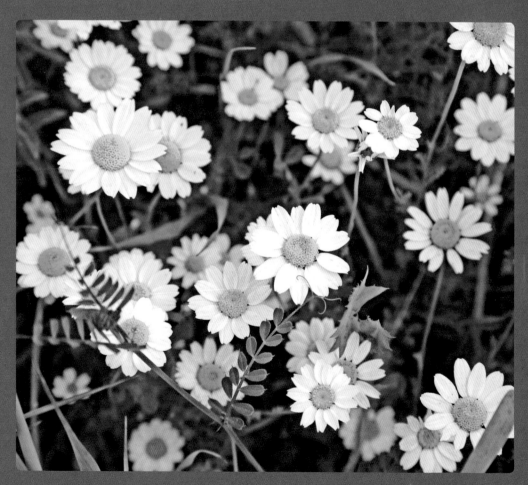

GROWING CHAMOMILE

Easily grown from seeds, chamomile is best cultivated by being sown directly in the garden in early spring. It prefers dry, light, well-drained soil but really isn't overly fussy. Rich soil produces larger and lusher foliage, but not necessarily more flowers. In fact, chamomile flowers are more prolific and more potent when grown in less-rich soil. Chamomile prefers full sun but enjoys cooler weather; it will get leggy and/or bolt in really hot weather. If you live in a hot area, sow very early in the spring so the flowers have an opportunity to bloom before the full heat of summer. In some areas, you can get two harvests, one in the early spring and another in the late fall.

When flowers are fully open and fragrant, use your fingers as a rake to harvest them, pulling them up between your fingers into a gathering basket. You'll find this technique far more efficient than collecting the small flowers individually. Commercial harvesters use real rakes, much like blueberry or cranberry rakes, to gather buckets of blossoms.

Chamomile is lovely planted near paths; when you brush up against it, it releases a delicious pineapple- or applelike fragrance. In days of old, chamomile was known as the "plants' physician," because it was said to cure whatever ailments the plants near it suffered. Chamomile remains a popular companion plant in the garden and is often planted near other plants to keep them healthy and disease free.

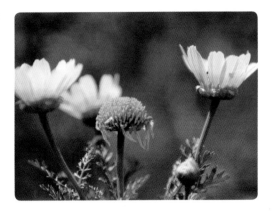

One of the best ways to pick the small, fragrant chamomile flowers is to use your fingers like a rake and gently comb through the plant, gathering several blossoms at a time.

MEDICINAL USES

Chamomile flowers have rich amounts of azulene, a volatile oil with a whole range of active principles that serve as anti-inflammatory and antifever agents, making it useful for treating arthritis and other inflammatory conditions. In one clinical study, 10 out of 12 people who drank chamomile tea instead of taking their regular pain medication at bedtime (for relieving general aches and pains, headaches, or arthritic pain) went into a deep, restful sleep within 10 minutes of retiring.

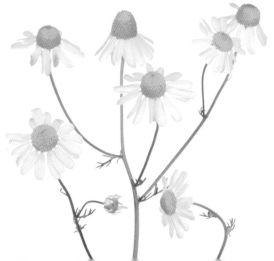

Other clinical studies confirm what herbalists have long known: this common wayside plant offers excellent support for the nervous and digestive systems. The flowers make a wonderfully calming tea that is good for easing stress and nervousness, promoting sleep, and aiding digestion. For infants and children, chamomile tea is a popular remedy for calming colic and childhood digestive issues. And the tea can be added to bathwater for a wonderfully relaxing and soothing bath. Chamomile also makes an excellent massage oil for relieving stress, anxiety, and muscle soreness.

Parts used

Primarily the flower, though the leaf can be useful as well

Key constituents

Azulene and other volatile oils, flavonoids, tannins, bitter glycosides, salicylates, coumarins, calcium, magnesium, phosphorus

Safety factor

Some people are allergic to chamomile. If you get itchy eyes or ears, a runny nose, a scratchy throat, or other signs of allergy, discontinue use.

Calming Chamomile Tea

Nothing could be simpler than making a cup of chamomile tea, whether with fresh or dried flowers, and few things are more calming and peaceful.

To make the tea:
Prepare an infusion of the flowers, following the instructions on page 29. Use 1 teaspoon of dried flowers or 2 teaspoons fresh flowers per cup of water, or 1 ounce of dried flowers or 2 ounces fresh flowers per quart of water. Let steep, covered, for 15 to 20 minutes. Chamomile contains bitters; the longer it steeps, the stronger the bitters. For a better-tasting, less bitter infusion, steep less.

To use:
Drink 2 to 3 cups daily, or as often as needed. This herb has lasting effects if used over a period of several weeks. It is nice to blend with other herbs that support the nervous system, such as lemon balm and rose petals, and it is excellent for infants and children as well as adults.

chamomile Eye Packs

These eye packs will help relieve eye stress and strain, dark circles, and puffiness.

To make the packs:
Place two chamomile tea bags in hot water and let sit for a couple of minutes, or until thoroughly saturated. Remove and let cool to a tolerable temperature.

To use:
Place a tea bag directly over each eye. Lie back and relax, leaving on the chamomile packs for 15 to 20 minutes.

Calming Herbal Bath for De-stressing

Immersing yourself in an herbal bath is much like stepping into a giant cup of tea: your pores open up, absorbing the healing properties of the herbs, and the warm water relaxes while it cleanses. It's healing at its finest.

To prepare the bath:
Mix together a handful each of dried chamomile blossoms, lemon balm leaves, and rose petals. Place the mixture in a large muslin bag, an extra-large tea strainer, or even an old nylon stocking. Attach directly to the faucet of the tub. Let hot water (the hottest possible) run through the herbs for a few minutes. Then adjust the water temperature to a comfortable level and fill the tub.

To use:
Dim the lights, light a candle, and immerse yourself in the calming essence of herbs. You might even want to enhance the relaxing effects on your nervous system by drinking a cup of warm chamomile tea.

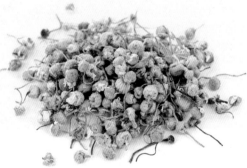

Chickweed / *Stellaria media*

Stellaria, chickweed's genus name, means "star," in reference to the plant's tiny white, starlike flowers. And chickweed is a star in the herb world. It can be found worldwide almost anywhere there's moist, cultivated soil — and yes, that means it's a frequent "weed" in gardens and yards. Don't discourage its growth or weed it all out. It's one of the best little weeds you can have in your garden. Shallow rooted, it provides living mulch for other garden plants. And when it comes time to gather greens for salad and herbs for medicine, chickweed will be readily available.

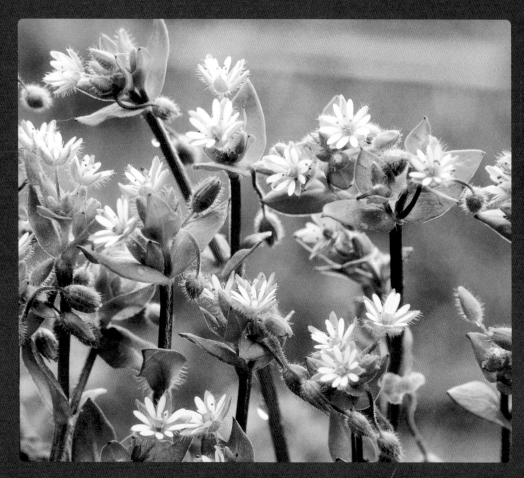

GROWING CHICKWEED

In truth, most people are trying to figure out how to get rid of chickweed in their gardens, rather than planting it. Chickweed is just one of those plants that show up in the garden and yard whether invited or not. A small, seemingly delicate annual, chickweed is hardier than it looks. It thrives in rich garden soil, easily reseeds, and prefers a sunny but cool location, though it will grow abundantly in partial shade as well. If you've not found chickweed in your garden and want to include it in your "wild medicinal weed patch," direct-sow the seeds in full sun or partial shade, water well, and watch for the tiny seedlings to sprout en masse. Chickweed can become a *bit* invasive, so beware. Eat regularly, juice, and use abundantly in your herbal remedies.

MEDICINAL USES

Don't be fooled by chickweed's seeming fragility. It is one of those mild-tasting plants that disguise their strength in sweetness. Chickweed is highly esteemed for its emollient, demulcent healing properties and is a major herb for addressing skin irritation, eye inflammation, and kidney and liver disorders. It makes an excellent poultice for treating hot, irritated rashes and skin problems. In a salve, chickweed has soothing, healing effects on the skin and is among the most effective remedies for relieving itchiness. It's often used to treat rashes, eczema, and nettle stings, and it's gentle enough to use on diaper rash and other skin irritations on infants and children.

Because it's gentle and soothing, chickweed is a well-known remedy for irritation

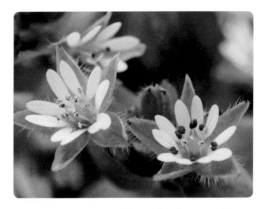

Stellaria media, chickweed's botanical name, means "little star," in reference to its small white flowers.

Part used
Aerial part

Key constituents
Vitamin C, calcium, potassium, phosphorus, iron, zinc, coumarins, saponins

Safety factor
Perfectly safe, with no known toxicity

and itchiness in the eyes. Used as poultice or pack, it cools and soothes the delicate membranes of the eyes.

The fresh, tender greens are a treasure trove of nutrients. They are delicious in salads and are also nice juiced or blended with pineapple juice. Due to their high nutritional value, mild diuretic action, and metabolism-stimulating properties, they are often found in weight-reducing formulas.

Chickweed doesn't dry or store well, so to preserve the fresh leaves for future use, it is best to tincture them, freeze, or convert them into a salve.

Chickweed Poultice

A chickweed poultice is another soothing remedy for irritated, itchy skin.

To make the poultice:
Mash a handful of fresh chickweed tops into a pulp, or place in the blender with a small amount of water (just a tablespoon or two per cup of fresh plant) and blend into a thick mash.

To use:
Fold the mashed herbs into a cloth and/or apply directly to the skin. Leave on for 30 minutes. Repeat with fresh herb as often as needed, until the itchiness and irritation cease.

Chickweed Super-Soothing Salve

This salve is useful for soothing irritated, dry skin and rashes. Use fresh chickweed if it's available, but fresh-wilt it (see page 37) after harvesting it to remove any extra moisture.

» Chickweed tops

» Oil

» Beeswax

To make the salve:
Infuse the chickweed in the oil, following the instructions on page 35. Use the resulting herbal oil and the beeswax to prepare a salve, following the instructions on page 38.

To use:
Apply as needed.

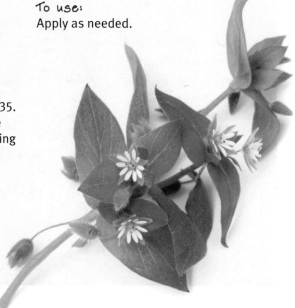

Dandelion / Taraxacum officinale

Half the world loves it, uses it for medicine, and dines on it regularly. The other half wages war on it with a heavy arsenal of pesticides, fungicides, and herbicides. Who's winning? Dandelion, for sure.

Dandelion's tenacity is part of its beauty and, perhaps, has something to do with its medicinal properties; it has the ability to thrive no matter what. Try as you might to banish this benign plant from farm fields and gardens, spunky dandelion returns year after year, seemingly undaunted, raising its golden rays to the sun each spring.

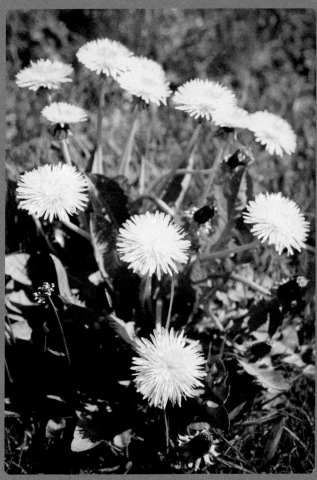

GROWING DANDELION

Dandelion is so hardy, so widespread, and so abundant that there's hardly reason to plant it. Just walk down the nearest country lane in the springtime, and you'll find entire fields filled with the bright blossoms of the dandelion (its name means "tooth of the lion"). Or let your lawn go unmowed, and within a few weeks you'll have a fresh crop of dandelion greens. But if for whatever reason you don't have a steady supply of fresh dandelion greens and roots, don't despair. Nothing could be easier to plant and grow. It's not fussy! Though it will grow just about anywhere, dandelion prefers rich, somewhat moist soil and full sun. Direct-sow seeds in the fall for early-spring greens. Greens can be harvested throughout the season, whether or not the plant is in flower. But the younger greens are definitely fresher, less bitter, and more tender. The roots can be harvested in late fall. Don't wait too long, however, as older roots get bitter and woody. If for no other reason, cultivate dandelion for the bees and other pollinators that love it!

MEDICINAL USES

The entire plant is useful as both medicine and food. The root is a classic liver tonic or "blood purifier," with a stimulating and decongesting effect on the liver. It also encourages optimal digestion, with a rich supply of bitter compounds that, having stimulated receptor sites on the tongue, signal the digestive tract: Get ready, food is coming! (The leaf has a similar effect.) The root also stimulates the production of bile, which in turn helps break down cholesterol and fat.

Parts used

Root, leaf, and flower

Key constituents

Vitamins A, B, C, and D; iron; potassium; calcium; inulin; sesquiterpenes; carotenoids

Safety factor

Some people are allergic to the milky latex of dandelion flowers and stems. If a rash should develop upon use of this latex, just discontinue the treatment.

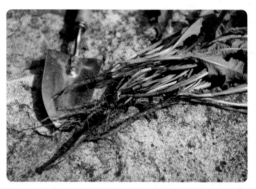

These dandelion roots are at the perfect stage for harvesting.

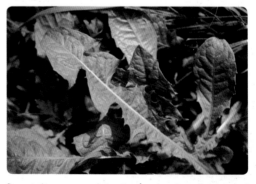

Dandelion greens taste best when harvested young, but they can be eaten anytime during the growing season.

Dandelion root has a mildly bitter flavor. When tender, the root can be chopped like a carrot and added to stir-fries and soups. The root is also delicious when sliced and pickled. Just use any pickling recipe for a surprisingly delightful flavor.

Dandelion leaf has long been used as a mild diuretic in cases of water retention and bladder or kidney problems. Unlike synthetic diuretics, however, dandelion leaf is a good source of potassium and replenishes rather than depletes this important nutrient. The leaf is also a good source of iron, calcium, vitamins, and a rich assortment of trace minerals. In fact, dandelion greens are a treasured food the world over. Throughout Europe and the Mediterranean, they are steamed, often with other wild greens, and served drizzled with olive oil and lemon juice.

Delicious! Add a few chunks of feta for a festive dandelion feast.

The leaves have a bitter zip to them; as cooked greens or tea, they are better when blended with milder herbs. My favorite way to eat the leaves is to steam them, then marinate them overnight in an Italian dressing with lots of honey. Oh, my! This is good. The dressing mellows the greens and removes a lot of the bitterness.

Even the flowers are food and medicine. You can make them into delicious dandelion wine or gently sauté them in butter for a fine crunchy flavor reminiscent of that of fried mushrooms. The flowers and stalks contain a milky latex that is helpful in getting rid of warts. It works, but you must be diligent; apply fresh latex directly on a wart several times daily for 2 to 3 weeks and watch the wart disappear.

Dandelion-Burdock Tincture for Liver Health

Dandelion and burdock root is an excellent and popular combination for cleansing and activating the liver. This tincture is useful in cases of poor or sluggish digestion, skin conditions such as acne and eczema, and any general health issue in which the liver might be of concern.

» 1 part burdock root
» 1 part dandelion root
» 80-proof alcohol, unpasteurized apple cider vinegar, or glycerin

To make the tincture:
Prepare a tincture of the roots, following the instructions on page 40.

To use:
Take ½ to 1 teaspoon three times a day.

HoRta foR LiveR and Kidney Health

A classic dish of wild greens, horta originated in Greece and is enjoyed throughout the Mediterranean. It generally consists of dandelion greens, nettles, purslane, and other common wild weeds. Though, of course, it can be enjoyed as a tasty accompaniment to any meal, horta can also be used medicinally to help people who have liver disorders, problems with digestion, and/or a congested liver. Easy to digest and very nourishing, it's a good meal when you're feeling depleted or worn out.

To make horta:
Gather fresh dandelion greens, nettles, purslane, and other wild greens as available. Steam for 5 to 8 minutes, or until the greens are well wilted. Drain, reserving the liquid for soup stock. Place the steamed herbs in a bowl and drizzle with olive oil and fresh lemon juice. If you like, crumble a bit of feta on top.

To use:
Though you can eat horta as often as you please, for medicinal purposes, eat ¼ to ½ cup two or three times daily.

Roasted Dandelion and ChicoRy Tea

Trying to cut back on coffee? Are the effects of too much caffeine each morning starting to wear? This tasty roasted dandelion and chicory tea won't have the stimulating effects of coffee, but it may help you to wean from your daily fix. Its flavor is bitter, dark, and rich, much like that of coffee. Try adding a bit of cream or half-and-half and a little honey to sweeten.

To make the tea blend:
Preheat the oven to 350°F. Slice or chop equal portions of fresh dandelion and chicory roots. Spread the roots evenly over a cookie sheet. Bake for 30 to 40 minutes, or until the roots are a dark brown. Let cool, then grind in an electric coffee grinder or blender. For added benefit, add ¼ to ½ part each of raw chicory and dandelion root.

To use:
Prepare a decoction of the roots, following the instructions on page 30. Drink ½ to 1 cup two or three times daily, or as desired.

Note: *You can also enjoy a New Orleans-style coffee by mixing ½ part Roasted Dandelion and Chicory Tea with ½ part coffee.*

Dandelion Mocha

Kami McBride, a community herbalist in northern California, has used her delicious roasted dandelion mocha blend to help hundreds of people successfully cut back on their coffee consumption. It's delicious and satisfying, with none of the irritating properties of caffeine.

» 3 tablespoons Roasted dandelion Root (see Roasting instructions on page 127)

» 1 tablespoon Raw cocoa nibs (or Raw chocolate)

» ½ cup milk or almond milk

» 1 tablespoon maple syRup or honey

» ½ teaspoon cinnamon powdeR

» ½ teaspoon vanilla extRact

» A dash of nutmeg or clove powdeR

To make the mocha:
Decoct the roasted dandelion root and cocoa nibs in 3 cups water, letting the mixture simmer for 30 minutes. Strain, then add the remaining ingredients, stir to combine, and reheat if necessary.

To use:
Drink as you please. If you want to cut down on your coffee consumption, try drinking Dandelion Mocha in place of coffee, perhaps mixing in a small amount of coffee so that you get a little of the buzz.

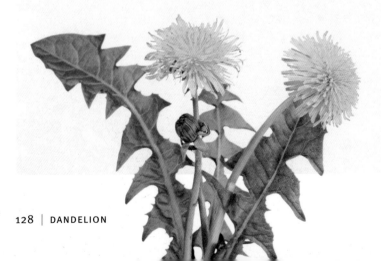

Echinacea is certainly one of the most popular herbs of our times, and for good reason. It is one of the top immune-enhancing herbs, helping to build immune-system strength and to fight off disease and infection. Many herbalists and natural-medicine practitioners feel it's the most important immune-enhancing herb in Western medicine. It is quite lovely, easy to grow, and hardy, and though incredibly effective, it is known to have few if any side effects or residual buildup in the body. What's not to like about this native plant? It's been called the "great herbal diplomat" because echinacea, perhaps more than any other medicinal plant, rescued herbalism from its twentieth-century obscurity.

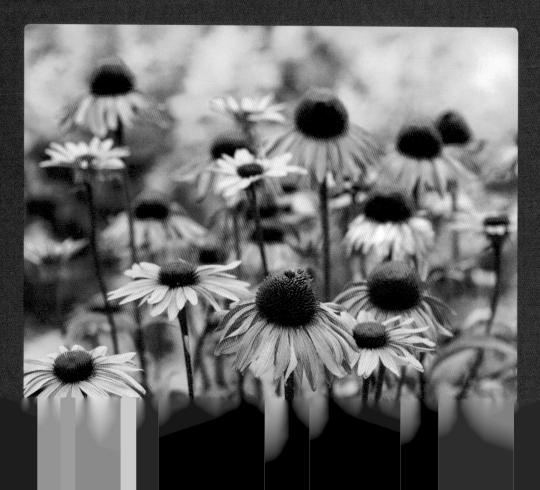

GROWING ECHINACEA

Echinacea shines in any garden. Commonly known as coneflower (*E. purpurea* is known as purple coneflower), it is easy to grow, unfussy, and strong and vigorous — perhaps a reflection of its immune-enhancing properties. Echinacea loves full sun and warm weather, though in very hot climates it may require partial shade. Think Appalachia, the prairies, and the Midwest, where echinacea is native. Its soil can be poor, though like most plants it will adapt and thrive as long as its most basic requirements are met. It can withstand drought, but it also does well on our mountain, where we are more often "drenched than droughted."

Parts used

Root, leaf, flower, and seed

Key constituents

Polysaccharides, caffeic acid, echinacoside, sesquiterpenes, tannins, linoleic acid, beta-carotene, vitamin C

Safety factor

Some people have allergic reactions to echinacea. If you get itchy eyes or ears, a runny nose, a scratchy throat, or other signs of allergy, discontinue use.

MEDICINAL USES

Extensive research, much of it conducted in Germany and other European countries, confirms that echinacea raises the body's natural resistance to infection by stimulating and aiding immune function. It works, in part, by increasing macrophage and T-cell activity, the body's first line of defense against foreign antigens. It's also rich in polysaccharides, which help protect cells against invasion by viruses and bacteria. And it has antifungal and antibacterial properties, making it an effective medicine against certain types of fungal and bacterial infections. Though potent, it is safe, with few side effects; even young children and the elderly can use it safely.

Echinacea is always more effective if taken at the early signs of illness, before the illness has the opportunity to "settle in." Echinacea is particularly effective against bronchial and respiratory infections, sore throat, and oral infections, and in any situation where the immune system needs fortifying. As a tea or tincture, echinacea can be taken at the first sign of a cold or flu to boost immune-system function. Take it in frequent small dosages (see page 46 for dosage instructions) for it to be effective at warding off illness.

Echinacea Spray for Sore Throats

This spray is cooling, refreshing, and healing for sore and/or infected throats.

» ¼ cup echinacea tincture

» ⅛ cup vegetable glycerin or honey

» ⅛ cup water

» 1–2 drops peppermint essential oil

To make the spray:
Mix together the echinacea tincture, glycerin, and water. Add the peppermint essential oil drop by drop until the spray has the right flavor for your taste. Pour into a spritzer bottle.

To use:
Spray directly into the back of the mouth, toward the throat, once every half hour or as often as needed.

CHOOSING AN ECHINACEA

Avoid wild-harvested echinacea unless you know and trust your source to be a responsible and ethical steward of wild populations. Because of the huge demand over the past 40 years, corresponding to growing concerns of immune issues worldwide, echinacea is being poached unmercifully from its wild habitats. Several species are already at risk or endangered. The good news is that most of the echinacea available these days comes from organically cultivated sources. Currently several medicinal varieties are available; I suggest *Echinacea purpurea* because it's easily grown, effective, and more common than the other species.

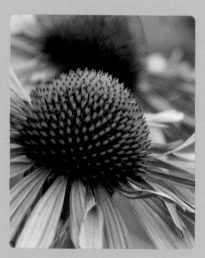

The beautiful flowers of Echinacea purpurea are not only medicinal, but a feast for the spirit as well.

Whole-Plant Echinacea Tincture

If you make only one tincture for winter, this should be it.

To make the tincture:

» *In the late spring*, gather fresh echinacea leaves, pack them loosely in a widemouthed glass quart jar, and add enough 80-proof alcohol (brandy, vodka, or gin) to cover by 2 to 3 inches. Place in a warm spot, and shake daily.

» *When the buds begin to ripen* on the echinacea plants, gather several young buds and add them to the jar with the echinacea leaves.

» *Later in the season*, when the flowers bloom (but before they are past their prime), gather several flowers and add them to the jar. Top off with alcohol, if necessary, so that it remains 2 to 3 inches above the plant material. If the jar is overfull, you can transfer its contents to a half-gallon widemouthed jar. Continue to shake daily.

» In fall, when the plants start to die back, their energy returns to the roots. On a late-fall afternoon, dig up an echinacea plant and harvest the roots. The plant should be 2 to 3 years old, which will make the root mature enough to have good medicinal potency but not too woody.

Clean the roots well, scrubbing, peeling, and breaking them apart as necessary. Then chop them into small pieces and add to the tincture jar, topping up the alcohol as necessary.

Let the tincture steep for 3 to 4 weeks. Strain, then bottle. A quart or more of whole-plant echinacea tincture should be enough to get you through a long winter.

To use:

For an acute situation, for example to ward off an infection, cold, or flu, take ½ teaspoon every hour. If this dosage doesn't seem to be working and you feel the immune system could use an additional boost, increase the dosage to ½ teaspoon every half hour. Decrease the dosage as you return to wellness.

To treat a chronic infection with echinacea, take ¼ to ½ teaspoon two or three times daily for 2 weeks. Discontinue for 1 to 2 weeks, then repeat the cycle as needed. While

I prefer a fresh whole-plant tincture, you can also make tincture from dried echinacea.

PLEASE NOTE: *Taking large amounts of echinacea for any length of time is not recommended, not because the plant is toxic but because it's generally not necessary and can even be counterproductive. High dosages are used only to mobilize the immune system to fight off the initial acute stages of infection. You should decrease the dose within 24 hours.*

DR. Kloss's Liniment

This, my absolute favorite liniment, is a formula handed down by a famous old herb doctor, Jethro Kloss, in his classic 1939 book, Back to Eden. *Dr. Kloss's liniment is useful both as a disinfectant and for inflammation of the muscles. I have been using this liniment for over 30 years and have found it to be absolutely the best disinfectant. Quite truthfully, you shouldn't be without it.*

>> 1 ounce echinacea Root powdeR
>> 1 ounce goldenseal Root powdeR (oRganically cultivated)
>> 1 ounce myRRh gum Resin powdeR
>> ¼ ounce cayenne powdeR
>> 1 pint Rubbing alcohol

To make the liniment:
Follow the directions for making a tincture. Because this liniment contains rubbing alcohol, be sure to label it EXTERNAL USE ONLY.

To use:
Either apply directly on wounds or use it to moisten a cotton ball and swab the infected area. Repeat as often as needed until the infection goes away.

"RegulaR" Echinacea TinctuRe

If you don't have a garden or the time to make a tincture from the whole plant, you can make a simple echinacea root tincture that will still be very effective — though perhaps not quite as effective as the whole plant tincture, simply because the different parts of the plant have different strengths of similar properties.

To make the tincture:
Prepare the tincture using fresh or dried echinacea root, following the instructions on page 40.

To use:
For an acute situation, take ¼ to ½ teaspoon every hour, or as often as needed. For chronic inflammation and infection, take ½ teaspoon three times daily for 2 weeks, then discontinue for 2 weeks (a rest period), and repeat the cycle as needed.

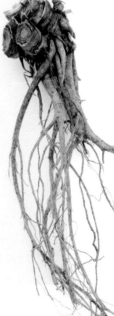

Elder / *Sambucus nigra*

Elderberry and elder flower are among Europe's most esteemed remedies for colds and flus. Travel through any European country in wintertime, and you'll find a variety of elder products lining pharmacy shelves. This large, handsome shrub has played an important role in the health and well-being of communities throughout history. In Old World tradition, an elder bush was commonly planted at the edge of the herb garden as the "protector" of the garden. Even its name, the *elder*, denotes its place of status in the garden. History aside, to

this day, elder flowers and berries are some of the best medicine and food we have and can be found growing in gardens and in the wild throughout most of temperate North America. It's prized not only by us two-leggeds; the tender tips are beloved by deer, moose, and other grazing animals, and more than 35 native birds are known to feast on the ripe berries in the summer. Plant it at the side of your garden, and watch the birds flock in.

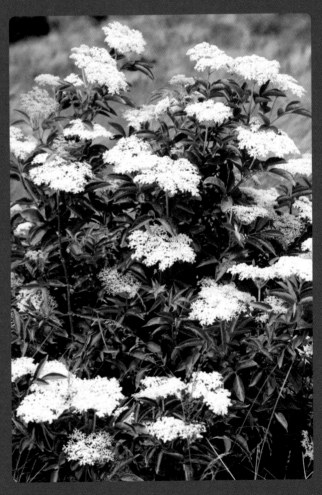

GROWING ELDER

A large perennial shrub that can reach upward of 30 feet, elder grows easily and quickly given the right conditions. It prefers moist, rich soil and partial shade to full sun. In the wild it's often found growing along stream banks and at the edges of farm fields, where there's water runoff and rich soil. It's said to be hardy to Zone 5, but I'm able to grow it even in Zone 3 due to the large amount of protective snow cover we get in the winter. It can be grown from seed, but it's challenging, and a cutting is an easier route for propagation. Be sure you have a large space to allow the elder to stretch out, or grow it at the edge of your garden or yard. Given the right conditions, it can be large!

MEDICINAL USES

Elder's beautiful lacy flowers are diaphoretic, meaning that they induce sweating, thereby helping to lower fevers. Elder's berries have immune-enhancing properties, and they're often combined with echinacea in immune-stimulating remedies for colds. The berries also have powerful antiviral properties and so are helpful in treating viral infections including flus, herpes, and shingles. They're also used for treating upper respiratory infections.

Elderberries make some of the best syrup (see recipe, page 138) and wine you'll ever taste. They also make great jams, jellies, and pies. The flowers are also edible and delicious. One of my favorite ways to eat them is in fritters, dipping the large, flat flower tops just as they're opening in a light batter, frying, and serving with elderberry jam. There are few things better!

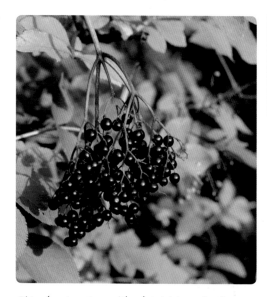

Elderberries hang like bright jewels from their branches in mid- to late summer. Leave some for the birds and wildlife to enjoy!

Parts used

Flower and berry

Key constituents

Vitamin C, vitamin A, bioflavonoids, flavonoids, phenolic compounds, beta-carotene, iron, potassium, phytosterols

Safety factor

Do not eat the raw (uncooked) berries in any great quantity, as they can cause digestive upset and diarrhea in some people.

Nutritive Tonic Berry-Good Tea

Yummy and delicious, these berries make an antioxidant-rich, heart-healthy tea that is delicious enough to drink on a daily basis.

» 2 parts dried elderberry
» 2 parts dried rose hip
» 1 part dried blueberry
» 1 part dried hawthorne berry
» Honey (optional)
» Lemon juice (optional)

To make the tea blend:
Combine the berries and rose hips. Infuse, using 1 tablespoon of tea blend per cup of water, following the instructions on page 29. Add honey and a bit of lemon juice, if desired.

To use:
Drink ½ to 1 cup once or twice daily to nourish the body and support heart health.

Nutritive Heart Tonic Tincture

The same berry mixture used in the preceding recipe — with the addition of heart-healthy linden blossom and hawthorn berry, leaf, and flower — makes a delicious and nutritious tincture for heart health. The tincture can be used safely and effectively with heart medication, as it's a tonic, not a "medicine" per se; it works through its nutritional component to strengthen the heart and circulatory system.

» 2 parts dried elderberry
» 2 parts linden flower
» 2 parts dried rose hip
» 1 part dried blueberry
» 1 part dried hawthorne berry, leaf, and flower
» 80-proof alcohol or unpasteurized apple cider vinegar

To make the tincture:
Follow the instructions on page 40.

To use:
Take ¼ to ½ teaspoon two or three times daily for 5 days, then discontinue for 2 days. Repeat the cycle for several weeks or even months.

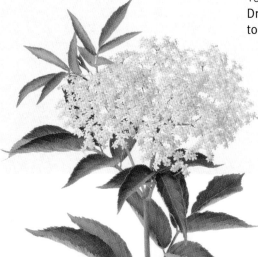

Gypsy Cold Care Remedy

This combination of herbs will help the body perspire, which will help lower a fever. The tea can also be used to treat allergies, hay fever, and sinus congestion.

» 1 part elder flower
» 1 part peppermint leaf
» 1 part yarrow flower and leaf

To make the tea blend:
Prepare an infusion of the herbs, following the instructions on page 29 and letting the herbs steep for 45 minutes, to make a very strong brew.

To use:
Sip throughout the day as needed.

Urinary Tonic Tea

This is a wonderful urinary tonic tea that can be helpful for those who are prone to urinary and bladder infections.

» 2 parts elder flower
» 1 part chickweed top
» 1 part dandelion leaf

To make the tea:
Prepare an infusion of the herbs, following the instructions on page 29.

To use:
Drink ½ to 1 cup once or twice daily to tone and nourish the urinary system.

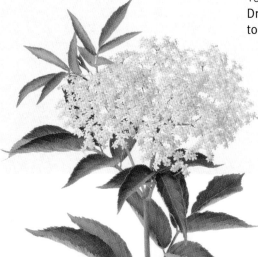

Elderberry Syrup

This may be one of the better elderberry syrup recipes on the planet. It's graciously shared by my friends Nancy and Michael Phillips, the authors of The Herbalist's Way. *Delicious enough to use just for sheer flavor alone, elderberry syrup is also helpful for warding off or speeding recovery from colds and flus.*

» 2 quarts fresh ripe elderberries

» ¼ ounce freshly grated gingerroot

» ½ teaspoon ground cloves

» Honey

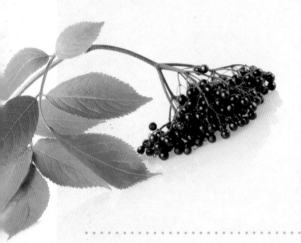

To make the syrup:

Combine the elderberries with ¼ cup of water in a large soup pot and simmer until soft. Strain out the pulp, reserving the liquid. Compost the solids and return the liquid to the pot. Add the ginger and cloves and simmer, uncovered, until the liquid reduces to about half its original volume. Pour the juice into a measuring cup and note its volume, then return to the pot. Add the same amount of honey and stir until thoroughly combined. Let cool, then bottle. Store in the refrigerator, and use within 12 weeks.

To use:

To treat or fight off a cold or flu, take 1 to 2 tablespoons several times throughout the day.

Variations

I've followed this recipe using dried elderberries, and the syrup has turned out, while not quite as delicious, still effective. Use 1 quart of dried berries with 2 quarts of water. Cook over low heat with the lid slightly ajar so that steam can escape, until the water is reduced by half. Strain, add the ginger and clove, and continue as above.

Adding elder flowers to the syrup introduces a diaphoretic property, helping you to "sweat out" a fever. After cooking down the juice with the ginger and cloves, you can turn off the heat, add ½ cup dried elder flowers to the hot juice, put the lid on, and let infuse for 20 minutes. Then strain the flowers from the syrup and proceed with the honey.

Goldenseal / *Hydrastis canadensis*

Goldenseal is quite possibly one of the most useful and valuable plants on the North American continent and one of North America's greatest contributions to world medicine. It was a popular medicinal herb among early Native American populations on the East Coast, and much of what we know of its uses comes from Native healers. With its infection-fighting alkaloids and bitters, goldenseal is powerful medicine, and it's one of the first herbs I turn to in cases of infection, whether internal or external. It can be used to treat a wide range of ailments, from skin infections to bronchial congestion and digestive complaints.

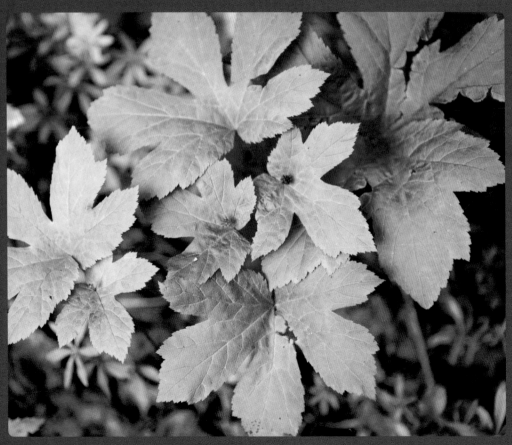

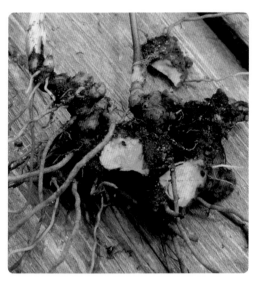

The small goldenseal rhizomes pack a mighty punch and are among our most potent native North American herbal remedies.

Parts used

Root and leaf (though the root is far more potent)

Key constituents

Hydrastine, berberine, resins, volatile oil, flavonoids, chlorogenic acid

Safety factor

If used internally over a long period of time (more than 3 to 4 weeks) or in excessive amounts, goldenseal becomes an irritant to the mucous membranes, causing inflammation. If you use it over the long term, use it for 3 weeks, take 1 week off, and then repeat the cycle. If mucosae become more irritated and inflamed when you use goldenseal, discontinue its use.

Because the herb is so effective and valuable, there is huge demand for it. Until recently little supply existed outside of wild populations, and as a result goldenseal is currently at risk in its native habitat. Thankfully, due to the dedicated work of United Plant Savers (see Resources) and other plant conservation groups, goldenseal is now being cultivated in fairly large quantities. When you purchase goldenseal, be sure to look for sources labeled ORGANICALLY CULTIVATED. Or grow it yourself. Please do not use wildcrafted goldenseal.

GROWING GOLDENSEAL

Goldenseal is a slow-growing perennial that has very specific habitat requirements. It grows naturally only in the shady hardwood forests of the eastern United States and Canada. Mimic the conditions of these forests as closely as possible and you'll generally have great success growing your own goldenseal patch. So, what are these requirements? Goldenseal loves humus-rich soil, a pH of 6 to 7, and at least 70 percent shade. If you have a large old maple, birch, or beech in your yard, then you probably can grow goldenseal under it. It will not do well under evergreens or oaks; they'll throw off the pH. Goldenseal is difficult to grow from seed. It can be done, but it requires stratification for up to 3 months. However, it is very easy to start from rhizomes. You can often divide a rhizome into smaller pieces; make sure that each piece has an "eye," or growing node. Plant in the fall 6 to 8 inches apart and about ½ inch deep. The root will be ready to harvest after 3 years of growth.

MEDICINAL USES

Goldenseal is considered a natural anti-biotic, and it is often paired with echinacea to help fight off infections, colds, and flus. It is particularly effective in treating infections of the mucous membranes, found in the respiratory, digestive, skin, and reproductive systems. It is a common ingredient in disinfectant washes for eye infections such as conjunctivitis, douches for vaginal infections (careful, it can be drying if not formulated correctly), mouthwashes for sore mouths and gums, and topical treatments for eczema and psoriasis. The root is often powdered for use in poultices for skin infections, abscesses, and wounds. And because of its rich bitter compounds, goldenseal is also helpful in treating liver, gallbladder, and digestive problems.

Beware! The root makes a *very* bitter tea; people generally prefer it in tincture or capsule form.

Goldenseal Salve

This salve has excellent disinfectant properties and is useful for treating skin infections and fungal infections such as athlete's foot.

- » 1 part chaparral leaf powder
- » 1 part goldenseal root powder (organically cultivated)
- » 1 part myrrh gum resin powder
- » Olive oil
- » Grated beeswax

To make the salve:
Infuse the herbs in oil, following the instructions on page 35. Add the beeswax to the oil, following the instructions on page 38, to turn it into a salve.

To use:
Apply a small dab directly to the infected area and gently massage into the skin. Repeat two or three times daily, or as needed.

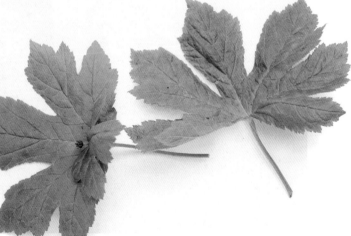

Goldenseal Wash for Eye Infections

This wash can be used to treat eye infections such as conjunctivitis.

» 1 teaspoon goldenseal root
(organically cultivated)

» 1 teaspoon marsh mallow
root or slippery elm bark

To make the wash:
Pour ½ cup boiling water over the herbs, cover, and let infuse for 45 minutes to 1 hour. Strain well; use a coffee filter or a very fine-mesh strainer lined with muslin. It's important not to have any particles of herb left in the wash. Bottle the liquid. Store in the refrigerator, where it will keep for 3 days.

To use:
You can use a specially made glass eyecup or simply a teaspoon that can be held firmly against the eye. Applying a cold tea is helpful for reducing swelling in the eye, but generally a warm tea feels better and is more soothing; you can warm the tea before use if desired.

Place approximately 1 tablespoon of the tea in the eyecup, hold firmly against an eye, and wash the eye thoroughly by blinking rapidly and/or holding the eye open and moving it from side to side, as if looking in each direction. Toss out the liquid, rinse out the eyecup, and repeat for the other eye.

Repeat three or four times daily for 3 or 4 days. If at any time the infection gets worse, discontinue treatment and call your health-care provider.

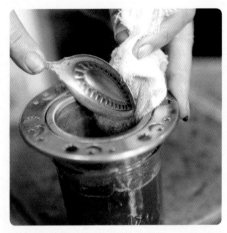

When making an eye wash, it's important to strain all of the herbal particles from the liquid.

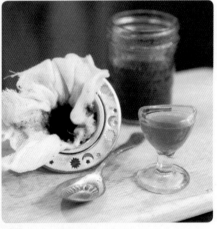

To use, pour the warm liquid into an eyecup or teaspoon and hold closely against the eye.

Goldenseal Clay Paste

Goldenseal clay paste is an excellent remedy for poison oak, poison ivy, and insect bites. I always keep a small jar of it on hand during the summer months, when biting insects abound. The goldenseal, clay, and salt are drying and drawing. The peppermint oil is cooling and takes away the burn and itch.

» 1 tablespoon goldenseal powder (organically cultivated)

» 1 tablespoon green or red clay

» 1 tablespoon Dr. Kloss's Liniment (optional; see recipe, page 133)

» ½ teaspoon sea salt (or Celtic or any other highly mineralized salt)

» 5-10 drops peppermint essential oil

To make the paste:
Combine the goldenseal, clay, liniment (if using), and salt with enough water to make a paste. Add the peppermint oil and stir well. Store in an airtight glass jar. The paste will keep for months; if it dries out while in storage, simply add a little water to reconstitute it.

To use:
Apply the clay paste directly to the affected area. The thickness of the paste will determine its drawing power. Generally a thin paste is all that's required, but if the rash or infection doesn't improve, use a thicker paste.

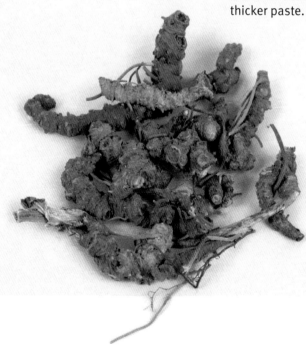

Hawthorn / *Crataegus laevigata*

The hawthorn tree brightens many a landscape around the world. When my grandmother came to this country from Armenia, she planted a hawthorn tree in the yard of each home she lived in. I have a descendant of one of those trees, a young sapling I dug from our childhood farm in northern California and brought to Vermont with me. Though not happy at first to be moved from a comfortable Zone 8 to a chilly Zone 3, it survived and now graces my yard.

Hawthorns are hardy and can live to upward of 200 years. Some are short and scraggly, some grow as thick hedgerows in the Irish and English countryside, some are stately old specimens found in the Italian countryside. In this country, many of the hawthorns you'll find are descendants of specimens our ancestors brought with them from the "old country." The berries are tasty and often enjoyed in syrups, jams, and jellies. They also make good medicine, as do the flower and leaf.

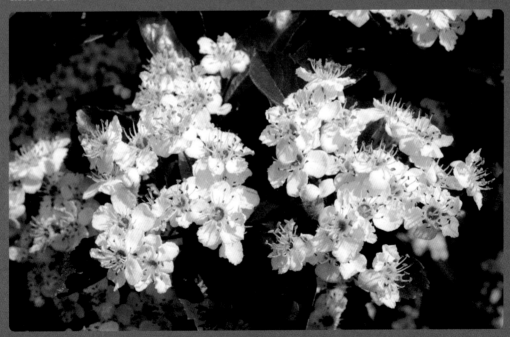

GROWING HAWTHORN

Hawthorn will tolerate a wide range of conditions and is quite easy to grow, but be careful to choose a species that fits the conditions of your own particular environment. And remember, it is a slow grower, but it can live to be more than 100 years old. Depending on the species, it can be small and shrubby or a large, elegant tree. It's a handsome tree, with clusters of white flowers in the spring and bright red berries (a favorite feast for birds) in the fall.

In general, hawthorn does well in full sun or partial shade at the edge of a forest or wooded area. It isn't overly fussy about soil pH, though given a choice it would choose rich, alkaline soil. Though you can usually find several varieties at nurseries, hawthorn self-sows readily, and it's easy to dig up the young saplings usually found in abundance beneath the mother tree to transplant to a new location.

MEDICINAL USES

Hawthorn is considered the herb supreme for the heart. The berries, leaves, and flowers are rich in bioflavonoids, antioxidants, and procyanidins, which feed and tone the heart. Hawthorn works in part by dilating the arteries and veins, enabling blood to flow more freely and releasing cardiovascular constrictions and blockages. It strengthens the heart muscle while helping to normalize and regulate blood pressure. It also helps maintain healthy cholesterol levels. Hawthorn is outstanding both to prevent heart problems and to treat high or low blood pressure, heart disease, edema, angina, and heart arrhythmia. (Because

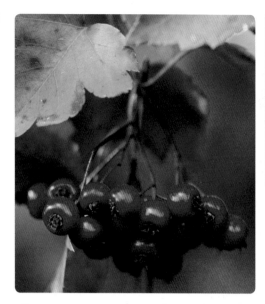

There are many varieties of hawthorn, all displaying clusters of bright red berries in late summer.

Parts used

Fruit, flower, leaf, and young twigs

Key constituents

Flavonoids, vitamin B, vitamin C, choline, acetylcholine, quercitin, triterpenoids, crategetin, rutin, procyanidin

Safety factor

Most naturopaths and herbalists feel that hawthorn preparations are safe to use in conjunction with allopathic heart medication, because hawthorn works through a nourishing and supportive mechanism, rather than druglike chemical changes. But if you're taking heart medication, check with your (hopefully open-minded) doctor before taking hawthorn or any other type of remedy, allopathic or herbal.

hawthorn doesn't store in the body and isn't accumulative in action, it's important to take hawthorn on a regular basis when using it as a heart tonic.)

Hawthorn also helps stabilize collagen and supports the health and repair of ligaments, tendons, and muscles. Hawthorn is excellent for strengthening the capillaries, which makes it useful for people who bruise easily. Try hawthorn tincture, tea, or capsules for 3 to 4 weeks and see if it helps reduce the amount of bruising.

The herb of the heart, hawthorn is also one of my favorite remedies for grief and deep sadness. Combine it with lemon balm, the milky tops of oats, and St. John's wort for a wonderful tea that helps alleviate the deep feelings of grief that often accompany loss.

Heartease Tea

This is an effective remedy for deep-seated grief and feelings of loss. It's also an effective remedy for seasonal affective disorder (SAD), when the lack of light during the long winter months brings on depression and lethargy.

» 2 parts hawthorn leaf, flower, and berry

» 1 part green oat top (milky top of just-ripening oats)

» 1 part lemon balm leaf

» 1 part St. John's wort flower and leaf

» Honey or stevia (optional)

To make the tea:
Prepare an infusion of the herbs, following the instructions on page 29. Sweeten with honey or stevia, if you like.

To use:
Drink 3 to 4 cups daily, until joy and hope again fill your heart.

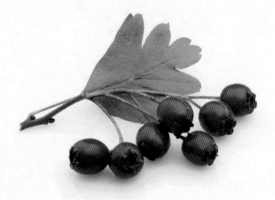

Sprinkles for the Heart

This delicious "sprinkle" is a heart-healthy flavoring for everything from hot and cold cereals and cinnamon toast to fruit salads and smoothies. Place it in a small bottle with a shaker top and set right on the table.

» 2 parts hawthorn berry powder

» 1 part cinnamon powder

» ½ part ginger root powder

» ⅛ part cardamom powder

To make the sprinkles
Mix the powders together, and store in a spice jar on the table.

To use:
Sprinkle on any plain fare that could use a boost of flavor.

Hawthorn Heart Balls

A delicious heart-healthy tonic.

» 2 parts hawthorn berry powder

» 1 part cinnamon powder

» 1 part linden flower powder

» ¼ part ginger root powder

» ⅛ part cardamom powder

» Honey or maple syrup (as a sweetener)

» Carob or cocoa powder (as a thickener)

To make the balls:
Follow the instructions for making herbal pills on page 43.

To use:
Take 1 or 2 pills daily.

Whole-Plant Hawthorn Tincture

For those who feel too busy to slow down for a cup of tea, hawthorn tincture is an excellent remedy, allowing them to take this nourishing, heart-healthy herb on a daily basis with minimal fuss.

To make the tincture:

» *In the spring*, gather fresh young hawthorn leaves, pack them loosely in a widemouthed glass quart jar, and add enough 80-proof alcohol (brandy, vodka, or gin) to cover them by 2 to 3 inches. Place in warm spot and shake daily.

» *Later in the season*, as soon as the flowers begin to open, collect a handful and add to the jar. Top up with more alcohol, if needed, to keep the liquid 2 to 3 inches above the plant material.

» *In the fall*, collect a handful of the ripe, bright red berries and add to the jar. Again, top up with alcohol if needed. Let the herbs macerate (infuse) in the alcohol for 4 to 6 weeks, shaking daily. Then strain and bottle the liquid.

To use:

As a heart tonic, take 1 teaspoon of tincture once or twice daily for 3 to 4 weeks. Discontinue for 1 week, then repeat the cycle.

Variation

Though I prefer using fresh hawthorn for tincturing, you can easily make a tincture from dried hawthorn leaves, flowers, and berries. Simply purchase them from a reliable source, place in a widemouthed quart jar, and cover with 80-proof alcohol.

Let sit in a warm, sunny spot for 4 to 6 weeks, shaking daily to potentiate and energize it. Strain and bottle the liquid.

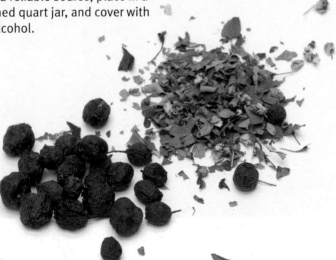

Lavender / *Lavandula officinalis, L. angustifolia*

What would the world be without lavender? It is, first and foremost, a beautiful, fragrant, and hardy plant that dresses up any garden space with its lovely lavender spikes and familiar aroma. Bees and butterflies as well as people flock to it wherever it grows. As if its beauty weren't enough, this lovely herb also has a wide range of medicinal uses and rates high on almost everyone's list of "essential herbs" to have on hand.

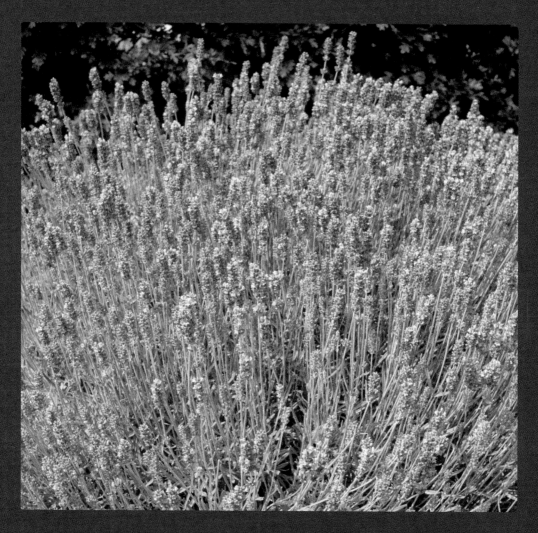

GROWING LAVENDER

Lavender is quite easy to grow in Zones 5 through 8 but needs a sunny, warm location and well-drained soil. Think southern France and the Mediterranean when you imagine lavender's natural environment. It will tolerate partial shade but loves full sunlight. It will tolerate cold but needs some winter protection in colder regions.

There's ongoing debate about which types of lavenders are most medicinal, and for what purposes. Generally, *L. officinalis* and *L. angustifolia* are highly regarded for their medicinal properties. I'm limited in what I can grow in my Zone 3 garden, but there are several lavender cultivars developed to thrive in colder regions — 'Hidcote,' 'Munstead,' and 'Grosso,' for example, which are said to be hardy to Zone 4. I have had good results growing both Hidcote and Munstead. They're not especially happy, but as long as we have sufficient snowfall to protect their roots, they come back each year. And while these cultivars may not be as highly regarded for their medicinal value as others, I have adapted to using what I have on hand in my garden.

If you have a green thumb or two, you could possibly germinate lavender from seed, but the attempt can be disappointing. Lavender can take several weeks to germinate, and then, if you're lucky, the germination rate is usually less than 50 percent. For beginners, I suggest getting three or four healthy plants from a local nursery. Once your plants are well established, you can take root divisions and cuttings to enlarge your lavender bed.

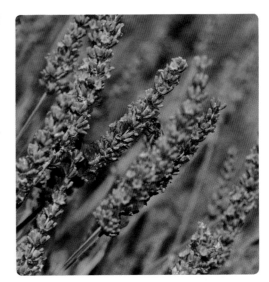

Lavender comes in many varieties. Each adds its own charm and beauty to the garden.

Lavender can grow quite large, depending on the species you're planting. Space plants at least 12 to 24 inches apart, or follow the recommendations for the specific species you're planting. The soil must be well drained and slightly sandy. A pH between 6.4 and 8 is ideal. Though lavender likes a good soaking occasionally, don't overwater it. Again, think Mediterranean: long, hot, sunny days, and only the occasional rain. And if temperatures drop below 20°F in your area, you may need to mulch your lavender plants to keep them alive through the winter.

For the highest quality, harvest lavender flowers when the buds are just starting to open. Most people wait too long. If you harvest the flowers when the buds are fully open, the medicinal properties won't be as strong and won't last as long.

MEDICINAL USES

Lavender has profound relaxing, calming, uplifting effects. It is a mild antidepressant, helpful in dispelling depression and melancholy. Combined with feverfew, it helps alleviate migraines and headaches. It is one of the best herbs to use in the bath to relieve tension, stress, and insomnia. After a long, stressful day, try a bath with a few drops of lavender essential oil, or a handful of lavender blossoms tied in a muslin bag, added to the water. You'll feel better immediately. Don't have time for a bath? Then rub 2 or 3 drops of lavender essential oil on your hands and massage the nape of your neck, your head, and your feet for calming relief. You can also make a calming massage oil by adding 8 to 10 drops of lavender essential oil to 4 ounces of vegetable or nut oil (grapeseed, almond, and apricot oil are lovely for this purpose).

Parts used

Flower primarily, but also the leaf

Key constituents

Flavonoids, linalool, eucalyptol, limonene, coumarins, tannins

Safety factor

Lavender is generally considered safe, though it's recommended that pregnant women avoid using it internally in large amounts.

An herb used traditionally to imbue courage and strength, lavender is still a favorite herb to strengthen the heart and mind in a stressful situation. Many women use it during childbirth. A drop or two of lavender essential oil rubbed directly on the feet and/or back of the birthing mother, or a warm poultice of lavender flowers held against her lower back, can bring gentle relief. Lavender is also one of the herbs used traditionally to bathe the new baby, welcoming him or her into the world. It seems an especially important ritual today, when children are so often alienated from the natural world.

Lavender's effectiveness as a traditional antibacterial, antifungal, and antiseptic agent has been confirmed by numerous clinical studies. It is useful in treating a host of infections, including staph, strep, colds, and flus. Alone or combined with tea tree oil, it can be applied directly to the skin to treat fungal infections such as ringworm and nail fungus, or it can be formulated in a douche to treat yeast infections. It is legendary as an herbal antiseptic and is used to disinfect and heal scrapes, wounds, and burns.

A popular antispasmodic, lavender is used in digestive formulas to relieve indigestion and is especially helpful for calming stomach muscle spasms, which are sometimes caused by irritable bowel syndrome and Crohn's disease.

Though lavender flowers are used in all manner of medicinal preparations, the essential oil of lavender is often referred to as "first aid in a bottle." This fragrant oil packs a mighty punch. It is one of the essential oils that I always carry with me when traveling, and I've found it useful in many situations. I've often added a few drops to a warm bath after a long day of travel. When my airplane is bouncing in the sky, I've quickly opened my small jar of lavender essential oil, breathed in deeply, and immediately felt calmer. I've used it to disinfect doorknobs and drinking glasses in areas where flu is rampant. I've seen it work wonders for painful burns, not only relieving the pain but also helping to disinfect and heal the wound. And its ability to take the pain out of a bee sting or insect bite is legendary.

Yes, I can get carried away in overt enthusiasm for these healing plants, but given lavender's successes over the centuries, it's hard not to join the crowd and applaud its many virtues.

Lavender Eye Pillow

These pillows have become quite popular for relieving eye strain, as well as for helping travelers and those who have trouble sleeping. They are wonderful if you have to fly the red-eye. I've been known to sleep the entire noisy night on the plane and wake refreshed as we land, with my lavender eye pillow still in place!

To make the pillow:
Cut a smooth soft piece of fabric (silk or soft cotton is ideal) in a rectangular shape approximately 10 inches by 5 inches. Stitch together on three sides, leaving one end open. Turn the fabric casing inside out, so the stitches are on the inside, and fill with dried lavender flowers. Don't overstuff, as you want the eye pillow to be able to follow the contour of your eyes.

You can add a drop or two of lavender essential oil to the pillow if you'd like a stronger scent, though generally the lavender flowers are scent enough. Then stitch the pillow closed.

To use:
Drape the pillow over your eyes, lie back, and relax. For added benefit, when at home you can heat your pillow in a warm oven or microwave (just be sure you don't burn it!) and place the warm pillow over your eyes or on your neck or lower back.

Lavender Antiseptic and Calming Spritzer

Lovely, calming, antiseptic, and safe! No wonder lavender spritzers are so popular.

» 7 tablespoons water

» 1 tablespoon vodka or witch hazel extract

» 5–10 drops lavender essential oil

» 1 (4-ounce) spritzer bottle

To make the spritzer:
Combine the water, vodka, and essential oil in the spritzer bottle.

To use:
Shake well before use, as the essential oil will have risen to the top. Use this lavender spritzer when you need a little calming essence. You can mist your car, your bedroom, the bathroom, or wherever. Lavender is also a powerful antiseptic. Use this spritzer as an antiseptic spray in bathrooms, in hotel rooms, and on your hands as needed.

Lavender-Lemon Balm Calming Aid

To calm nervous stress, try this relaxing tea. It is particularly delicious served iced or at room temperature.

To make the tea:
Brew 1 quart of extra-strong lavender tea and 1 quart of extra-strong lemon balm tea, following the instructions for making an infusion on page 29. Make up 2 quarts of fresh lemonade (lemons, honey, and water to taste). Combine the lemonade with the teas and stir well.

To use:
Drink as much and as often as needed.

Lavender-Feverfew Migraine Tincture

The poppy is optional but recommended. California poppy seed, leaf, and flower are better, but if you can't obtain them, any variety of poppy seed will work.

» 1 part California poppy
  (seed, leaf, and flower)
  or poppy seed (optional)

» 1 part feverfew leaf

» 1 part lavender bud

» 80-proof alcohol, unpasteurized
  apple cider vinegar, or glycerin

To make the tincture:
Follow the instructions on page 40.

To use:
For long-term use for frequent migraine headaches, take ½ teaspoon two times a day for up to 3 months. Discontinue for 3 to 4 weeks, and then repeat the cycle as needed. For acute situations (at the onset of a migraine or headache), take ¼ teaspoon every 20 to 30 minutes for up to 2 hours.

Note: *Women should discontinue use of this tincture during menstruation, as it can stimulate bleeding. In fact, feverfew is sometimes used to bring on a delayed menstrual cycle.*

HEADACHE RELIEF

The next time you have a headache, try an old-fashioned remedy: Take several drops of migrane tincture and then treat your feet to a hot lavender footbath (add a few drops of lavender essential oil to hot water), rub a drop or two of lavender essential oil on the nape of your neck and massage it in, and then hold a lavender eye pillow (see page 152) over your eyes for 10 to 15 minutes. Better yet, get a friend to massage your feet with lavender massage oil (see page 155) while you rest comfortably on the couch with your warm lavender eye pillow in place.

Calming Lavender Massage Oil

It's quick and easy to make lavender massage oil by just adding the essential oil to a "fixed oil" (the technical term for a vegetable, nut, or seed oil, distinguishing it from the steam-distilled "essential" or "volatile" oils of a plant). But for greater medicinal benefit, use lavender flowers as well.

» 1½ ounces dried lavender buds

» 4 ounces vegetable, nut, or seed oil (apricot kernel, almond, grapeseed, or a combination)

» 5–10 drops lavender essential oil

To make the massage oil:
Place the lavender buds in a wide-mouthed glass quart jar. Pour the oil over the buds, put on the lid, and let sit in a warm, sunny spot for 2 to 3 weeks. (Alternatively, you can hasten the process by gently warming the oil and buds in a double boiler for 45 minutes to 1 hour.) Strain the buds from the oil and add the essential oil drop by drop, until the scent is to your liking. Bottle and store in a cool spot out of direct sunlight, where the oil will keep for at least 6 months.

To use:
Keep a small bottle by your bedside to use for evening massages and a small bottle in your bathing area for a calming massage and/or body oil after a hot bath.

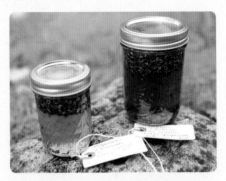

The dried lavender blossoms in this massage oil are allowed to steep for 2 to 3 weeks.

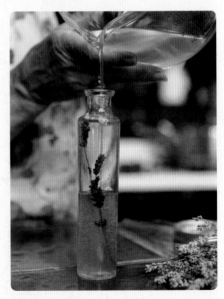

For a sweet touch, add a sprig or two of dried lavender to the bottle of finished oil.

Lemon Balm / *Melissa officinalis*

Rare is the plant that is so delicious and so effective a remedial agent. Lemon balm's species name, *officinalis*, indicates that the plant has long been an "official" herb of apothecaries. Its genus name, *Melissa*, derives from *melisso-phyllon*, a Greek term meaning "bee leaf." Anyone who has grown lemon balm knows that bees are very attracted to this plant; it fairly hums with bee activity. Camouflaging its potent medicinal actions in sweet-scented leaves, lemon balm is considered one of the most important members of the large mint family. It is a featured remedy for heart disease (and heartache), depression and anxiety, nervous disorders, and a host of viral and bacterial infections.

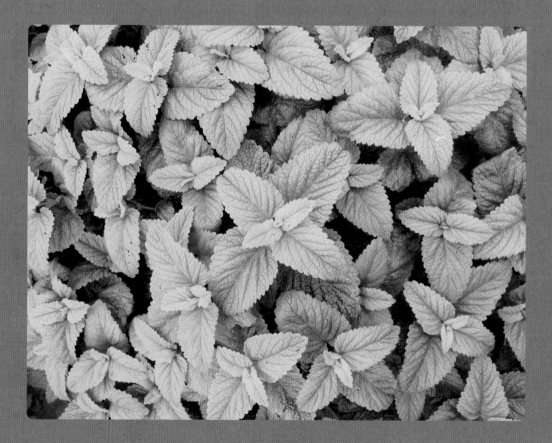

GROWING LEMON BALM

Lemon balm is a fast-growing perennial hardy to Zones 4 through 9, and it can be grown as an annual in colder regions. It self-sows easily, so once you have a few plants established, it should build its own bed without much fuss. Lemon balm prefers moist but well-drained soil and a bit of shade, though it will do nicely in full sun as well. Sow seeds directly in the soil in fall or start seeds indoors in spring.

Lemon balm always makes quite an impression on garden visitors, not due to a striking appearance or stunning flowers (it's rather plain on both accounts) but due to its irresistible fragrance and flavor. Plant it where visitors can easily brush up against it or reach out to nibble its tasty leaves. Lemon balm leaves can be harvested anytime during the growing season but are more flavorful before the plants flower. And when plants do begin to flower, you can snip them back for a second crop of leaves. The leaves retain their wonderful scent even when dried. (For drying instructions, see page 19.)

MEDICINAL USES

"Balm is sovereign for the brain, strengthening the memory and powerfully chasing away melancholy," wrote John Evelyn, a well-known herbalist, in the 1600s. Paracelsus called lemon balm the "elixir of life," a rather high title, and Dioscorides used it for "sweetening the spirit." It's intriguing how often the rich and lively history of herbs is supported by modern science. As for lemon balm, modern studies have shown that lemon balm's rich concentration of volatile

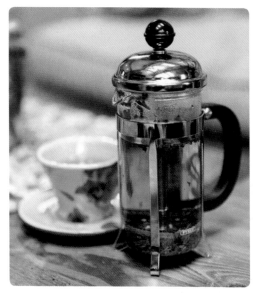

A French press is excellent for infusing herbal tea.

Part used

Aerial part of the plant; the leaf is rich in essential oil

Key constituents

Citral, citronellal, tannins, bitters, polyphenols, vitamin C, calcium, magnesium, catechin, resins, flavonoids

Safety factor

Lemon balm is considered a thyroid inhibitor; those suffering from hypothyroidism or low thyroid activity should use it only under the guidance of a health-care practitioner.

oils, specifically citral and citronellal, calms the nervous and digestive systems, with antispasmodic actions. A tea made of lemon balm and chamomile is an excellent remedy for stomach distress and nervous exhaustion. It also functions as a mild sedative, especially helpful for insomnia caused by grief and sadness; blend lemon balm with passionflower and a small amount of lavender buds and drink a cup or two a couple of hours before bedtime.

Lemon balm is high on the list of herbs commonly used to treat heartache and depression. I use it in Heartease Tea (page 146), which combines lemon balm with St. John's wort, oats, and hawthorn (berry, flower, and leaf) in a delicious tea that helps bring a ray of light and sweet hope to the grieving heart. The tea is also an effective remedy for seasonal affective disorder (SAD).

Lemon balm is a beloved herb for children. It can calm a restless child and is a known aid for ADD and ADHD. It's also helpful for soothing children with recurring nightmares; just give a small dose before bedtime. Even more helpful is a warm chamomile bath followed by a gentle lavender oil massage and a tablespoon of lemon balm glycerite (tincture made with glycerin) just before bedtime.

In addition to its soothing and calming properties, lemon balm is rich in polyphenols, which have a strong antiviral action. This explains, at least partially, its effectiveness against herpes and shingles. Herbalists often combine lemon balm with licorice to create a particularly effective remedy against the virulent herpes virus.

Because it's so delicious, lemon balm is often prepared as tea, but is it also tasty as a culinary herb. Add a few of the flavorful leaves to salads, soups, grain dishes, and smoothies for a refreshing lemony flavor. Lemon balm also makes one of the tastiest tinctures. Try a glycerin tincture of lemon balm; it will sweeten anyone's heart.

LEMON BALM FOR LONG LIFE

One of my dearest elder friends and herbal teachers, Adele Dawson, was a great fan of lemon balm and grew copious amounts of it in her wild gardens. When I came to visit with my herbal students, she would greet us at her doorstep with a tray full of gleaming green glasses filled with her favorite daily "remedy": Combine a handful of lemon balm leaves, a few borage leaves, thinly sliced lemon and orange, a shot of cognac, half a cup of honey, a bottle of claret, and a pint of seltzer water. Let stand with enough ice to cool, strain, and decorate with the blue, star-shaped blossoms of borage.

Adele lived well into her 90s, following in the footsteps of Llewelyn, the thirteenth-century prince of Glamorgan, who drank lemon balm tea every day and purportedly lived to the age of 108.

Carmelite Water

First made by the Carmelite nuns in the seventeenth century, Carmelite water was once a secret formula based on lemon balm. Many versions are sold today — some of which don't even contain lemon balm. Carmelite water is used as a digestive aid and mild tonic.

» 3 parts lemon balm leaf
» 1 part angelica root
» ½ part coriander seed
» ½ part lemon peel
» ¼ part nutmeg
» 80-proof brandy
» Honey (optional)

To make the water:
Tincture the herbs in the brandy, following the instructions on page 40. If desired, before bottling add ¼ cup of warmed honey per quart of tincture and stir to combine.

To use:
Drink a small shot glass full before dinner as a relaxing herbal aperitif and digestive aid.

Colic Remedy

Actually, this tea is helpful for anyone with digestive disturbances due to nervous stress, but it is especially helpful for infants and for those elders who have stomach problems.

» 3 parts lemon balm leaf
» 2 parts chamomile flower
» 1 part dill seed and leaf

To make the tea:
Prepare the herbs as an infusion, following the instructions on page 29.

To use:
For infants with colic, give 1 to 2 teaspoons of the tea before nursing or feeding. For adults, drink as needed.

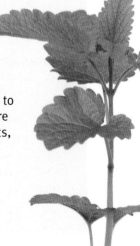

Lemon Balm Glycerite

Wonderfully relaxing and calming. It is probably the most delicious tincture you'll ever taste! It's almost cordial-like in flavor and could be served as an after-dinner drink, but because it's nonalcoholic, it's great for children and people who prefer not to use alcohol-based products.

To make the glycerite:
Fill a widemouthed glass jar with lemon balm leaves. Prepare a solution of 3 parts glycerin and 1 part water. Fill the jar with the solution. Cover, then let the jar sit in a warm spot for 3 to 4 weeks. Strain and bottle the liquid. Store at room temperature, where the glycerite will keep for at least several months.

To use:
For adults, take ½ to 1 teaspoon as needed. For children, adjust the dose according to size and weight; see the dosage chart on page 48.

Lemon Balm Bath

Both relaxing and stimulating, this bath is used for dispelling "negative energy," lifting the spirits, and just good old bathtime fun.

>> 2 parts fresh or dried lemon balm leaf

>> 1 part chamomile flower

>> 1 part lavender bud

>> 1 part rose petal

To prepare the bath:
Mix together the herbs. Tie ½ cup or more of the herb mixture into a large cloth bag, an extra-large strainer, or even an old nylon stocking. Fasten to the faucet of the tub. Let hot water (the hottest possible) run through the herbs for a few minutes. Then remove the herbs and fill the bath, adjusting the water temperature to a comfortable level.

To use:
Soak in the bath for at least 30 minutes. If you tied the herbs in a cloth bag, use it to gently massage your body. Step out, dry, and complete this healing treatment with a gentle massage using lavender massage oil (see page 155).

Licorice / *Glycyrrhiza glabra*

The sweet constituents of licorice root have made it a well-known and popular candy for generations. And it's no wonder; licorice is 50 times sweeter than table sugar! But it's glycyrrhizic *acid*, not a sugar, that makes licorice so sweet tasting. Glycyrrhizic acid is also responsible, in part, for licorice's amazing medicinal properties. When broken down by the stomach, glycyrrhizic acid yields anti-inflammatory and antiarthritic properties that act similarly to hydrocortisone and corticosteroids in the body. Of course, it's never as simple as one chemical doing it all; otherwise, we'd call it a drug, not an herb. Licorice works through a complex combination of constituents including mucilaginous material that make it soothing for inflamed and irritated tissue, phytohormones that aid human hormones by providing "building blocks" for the endocrine system, and antiviral agents that effectively ward off infections such as herpes and shingles.

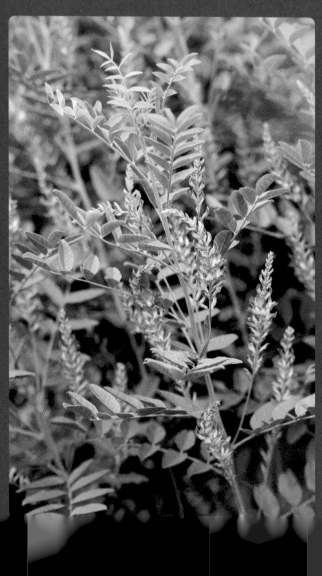

GROWING LICORICE

Licorice is most often regarded as a tender perennial, hardy in Zones 7 to 10. I have a couple of fairly healthy licorice plants growing in my own gardens in Zone 3, which shows it can be done, but they are surviving, not thriving. Generally speaking, licorice is another "Mediterrean medicinal plant" that prefers hot weather and full sun or partial shade. It prefers a slightly sandy soil, with a pH between 6 and 8. Like all members of the Leguminosae family, licorice "fixes," or sets, nitrogen in the soil. Seeds germinate well and quickly and plants grow to be quite large and handsome. Space plants 1½ to 2 feet apart in a sunny spot in the garden. Keep the soil moist until the seeds have germinated and young plants are well established. Licorice needs a few years of growth to develop its full medicinal potential. Harvest roots in the fall of the third or fourth year. (After the fourth year, the roots tend to become woody and tough.) Slice or chop the fresh roots, dry them (see instructions, page 19), and store in an airtight glass jar.

MEDICINAL USES

One of the most renowned herbal medicines in history, licorice is employed in many parts of the world for its demulcent, antiviral, and anti-inflammatory properties. It is the herb of choice for soothing irritated and inflamed tissue such as in cases of sore throat, bronchial inflammation, and stomach and bowel irritation. It is very helpful for both gastric and peptic ulcers. My grandmother's favorite remedy for stomach

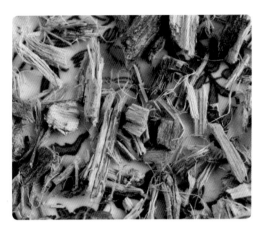

The natural sweetness of licorice root adds flavor to less tasty herbal teas.

Part used

Root

Key constituents

Glycyrrhizic acid (also known as glycyrrhic acid), phytoestrogens, coumarins, flavonoids, essential oil, polysaccharides

Safety factor

Glycyrrhizic acid can cause sodium retention and potassium loss, resulting in stress to the heart and kidneys. Individuals with a history of high blood pressure, water retention, heart palpitations, and other signs of heart and/or kidney stress should use licorice only under the guidance of a qualified health-care practitioner.

ulcers was fresh-juiced cabbage leaves and licorice root tea, with which she cured her own gastric ulcer when she was in her 80s.

Licorice tea and tincture are excellent for toning and strengthening the endocrine-gland system and are a specific remedy for adrenal exhaustion. Most menopausal women (and some men) could stand to have their adrenal glands nourished with licorice. Licorice gently supports the adrenal glands' ability to produce hormones and aids in the breakdown and elimination of excess or "worn-out" hormones via the liver and kidneys.

Licorice is often considered to be estrogenic or estrogen stimulating. Of course, plants contain not human hormones but phytohormones, or plant hormones that provide the building blocks the body uses to produce human hormones. In essence, licorice root may help the body produce more estrogen, but only by providing essential nutrients that the liver and endocrine system need to produce hormones and generally only if your system needs estrogen.

Licorice has a long history of use for relieving throat inflammation and for strengthening the vocal cords. It has a thick, sweet flavor, which makes it a nice addition to tea in small amounts. Surprisingly, the root can be almost too sweet, and some people find its flavor rather offensive when it's brewed by itself. To increase its palatability, try blending licorice with other herbs in syrups, teas, and tinctures. You can also just eat the licorice root "straight up" (the dried or fresh whole root). Children, especially, enjoy chewing on licorice sticks.

Gentle LicoRice Laxative

Licorice has mild laxative properties and is at the same time healing to irritated bowel membranes. For mild and/or occasional constipation, try this formula. (If needed, you can increase the yellow dock portion for a stronger laxative effect.)

» 1 paRt chopped dandelion Root
» 1 paRt chopped licoRice Root
» ½ paRt chopped yellow dock Root

To make the laxative:
Combine the roots and mix well. Prepare as a decoction, following the instructions on page 30, using 1 to 2 teaspoons per cup of water.

To use:
Drink a cup or two as needed. If stronger action is required, increase the yellow dock root or add ½ part cascara sagrada.

Adrenal Tonic Tincture

Licorice is one of the best tonics for adrenal exhaustion. Try this formula if you frequently feel tired and exhausted and life has lost its zest.

» 1 part chopped licorice root

» 1 part chopped Rhodiola root

» 1 part chopped Siberian ginseng

» ½ part chopped cinnamon bark or gingerroot

» 80-proof alcohol

» Honey (optional)

To make the tincture:
Tincture the herbs in the alcohol, following the instructions on page 40. Before bottling, add ¼ cup of warmed honey per quart of tincture and stir to combine.

To use:
Take ½ to 1 teaspoon three times daily for 3 months. Discontinue use for 1 month, then repeat the cycle as needed.

Licorice-Ginger Balls

A tasty and soothing recipe for singers and those with sore throats.

» 2 tablespoons licorice root powder

» 1 teaspoon gingerroot powder

» Honey

» Cinnamon or cocoa powder (as a thickener)

To make the balls:
Make herbal pills, following the instructions on page 43, using honey and a drop or two of water to form the paste and cinnamon or cocoa powder as a thickener.

To use:
Take 1 or 2 balls as needed.

LicoRice Cough SyRup

This syrup is delicious, sweet, and particularly effective for soothing irritated membranes, such as in cases of sore throat, coughs, and laryngitis.

» 1 paRt chopped licoRice Root
» 1 paRt mullein leaf
» 1 paRt wild cheRRy baRk
» Honey oR otheR sweeteneR

To make the syRup:
Follow the instructions for making a syrup on page 33.

To use:
Take ½ to 1 teaspoon every half hour or as needed.

Soothing ThRoat Balls

These pills work wonders for sore throat, laryngitis, and other infections of the throat or mouth.

» 2 paRts licoRice Root powdeR
» 1 paRt echinacea Root powdeR
» 1 paRt goldenseal Root powdeR (oRganically cultivated)
» 1 paRt maRsh mallow Root powdeR
» Honey
» A few dRops of peppeRmint essential oil
» CaRob powdeR (as a thickeneR)

To make the balls:
Follow the instructions for making herbal pills on page 43. Feel free to adjust the flavors to suit your taste.

To use:
Take 1 or 2 pills daily for best results.

Marsh mallow belongs to the large and benevolent mallow family, which also includes hollyhock, okra, and a variety of interesting medicinal plants. Few if any mallows are toxic — it's a nice family to have in the neighborhood. Most are sweet and delicious, demulcent and emollient (soothing internally and externally), and useful as both food and medicine.

Long before marsh mallow became known and respected as a medicinal plant, it was valued as a delicious root vegetable. Romans, Greeks, and other ancient peoples were known to feast on it. The French turned marsh mallow the plant into marshmallow the confection. They cooked the gummy juices of the roots with eggs and sugar, then whipped the mixture until light and airy. This thick, sweet, mucilaginous confection was popular for soothing coughs and calming digestive upset in babies. Over time, the plant extracts were replaced with gelatin and the sugar with corn syrup, and confection metamorphosed into the familiar gummy white marshmallow now synonymous with campfires and cookouts. The original marsh mallow and its modern-day counterpart bear little resemblance, other than a shared common name.

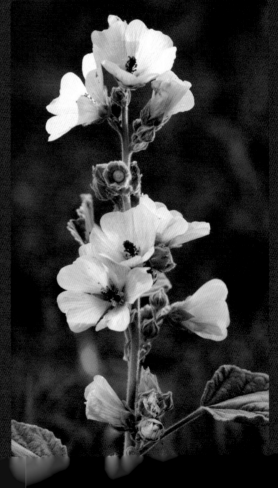

GROWING MARSH MALLOW

Marsh mallow is a quick-growing perennial handsomely adorned with soft gray-green leaves and lovely pink flowers. It is not fussy, and once established it will grow readily and easily. Give it lots of space, as it grows quite large (upward of 4 feet). Taking its name from its natural habitat, marsh mallow gravitates to marshy, damp areas. It will grow well in full sun or partial shade; prefers loamy, moist soil; and needs light to moderate watering. It prefers a moderate climate (Zones 5 to 8), but I am able to grow it in Zone 3 due to our thick snow coverage, which shelters the plant's roots through the winter. Though seeds germinate quickly and fairly reliably, they have to be stratified (chilled in winterlike conditions) first. Beginners may have better luck starting with one or two young plants purchased from a nursery. Be sure to purchase *Althaea officinalis*, as there are many varieties of malvas but marsh mallow is the most medicinal.

Parts used

Root primarily, though the leaf and flower are also used

Key constituents

Polysaccharides, flavonoids, betaine, coumarins, beta-carotene, vitamin B, calcium

Safety factor

Marsh mallow is a perfectly benign herb with a long record of safe use among those who know its virtues!

MEDICINAL USES

Marsh mallow root is more than 11 percent mucilage and 37 percent starch, making it an exceptionally rich, nutritive tonic. The root's large sugar molecules swell upon contact with water, creating the sweet mucilaginous gel that marsh mallow is so famous for. Because of its sweet flavor and its rich mucilaginous properties, marsh mallow is a popular medicine for soothing all manner of inflamed tissue. It is specific for treating inflamed and irritated tissues of the respiratory system, digestive system, and skin, and particularly useful for soothing irritation and inflammation in the bowel. It is probably most well known for its soothing actions on the bladder and kidneys and is an important ingredient in many formulas for treating bladder and kidney infections. And it is helps neutralize excess acid in the stomach, making it useful in cases of stomach ulcer.

While marsh mallow root may not have exceptional antiviral, antibacterial, or other infection-fighting properties, its soothing, demulcent action makes it an excellent aid for dry coughs, as it lubricates and moisturizes the lungs. It is also often combined with more-aggressive and/or irritating herbs to mellow their effects.

Externally, marsh mallow is soothing to the skin. A paste of marsh mallow mixed with chamomile tea or water makes an excellent poultice for moisturizing dry, chapped skin. Marsh mallow is also effective in the bath for soothing itchy, dry skin, including eczema. And marsh mallow is good for keeping babies' bums soft and dry (see the recipe on page 169).

Herbal Capsules for Bladder Infection

This is one of my favorite recipes for treating bladder infection. Taken with cranberry juice and/or berries, this formula is very effective and will cure all but the most tenacious cases of bladder infection.

» 2 parts uva ursi leaf powder

» 1 part echinacea root powder

» 1 part goldenseal root powder (organically cultivated)

» 1 part marsh mallow root powder

» "00" gelatin or vegetable capsules

To make the capsules:
Combine the powders and mix well. Encapsulate in "00" capsules. Store in an airtight glass jar.

To use:
Take 2 capsules every 3 to 4 hours until the bladder infection subsides. If the infection doesn't improve within a few days, seek the advice of your health-care practitioner. Drink plenty of water and unsweetened cranberry juice for added protection and healing.

Variation

If you're prone to bladder infections, you might benefit from preparing this formula as a tincture, which will penetrate the bloodstream more quickly. Take ½ to 1 teaspoon of the tincture at the first signs of an infection; this is often enough to fight it off.

MARSH MALLOW VS. SLIPPERY ELM

At one time slippery elm was the "mucilage of choice" in North America. But since elm trees, including the slippery elm, were decimated by Dutch elm disease, for ethical and environmental reasons most herbalists and conscious consumers prefer marsh mallow. Because marsh mallow is a fast-growing perennial, whereas slippery elm is a slow-growing and endangered tree, it only makes sense to use marsh mallow in place of slippery elm whenever and as much as possible.

Marsh Mallow Baby Powder

This makes an excellent all-natural, safe, and effective powder for treating and preventing diaper rash.

- » 1 part arrowroot powder
- » 1 part cornstarch
- » 1 part marsh mallow root powder
- » 1–2 drops lavender essential oil

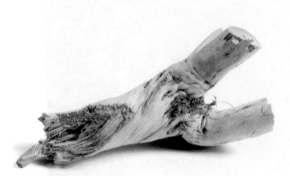

To make the powder:
Mix the powders together in a large bowl (a wire whisk works well for this). Add a drop or two of lavender essential oil and whisk in well. Cover with a thick cotton towel and let sit overnight in a dry room; this allows the oil and powder to dry. Whisk again and package in a powder container for easy application.

To use:
Sprinkle over the baby's bottom as needed to absorb excess moisture.

Urinary Tonic for Bladder Health

This is a soothing, healing remedy for bladder irritation — not quite a full-blown infection, but rather a low-grade, chronic irritation.

- » 1 part chickweed top
- » 1 part dandelion leaf
- » 1 part marsh mallow root
- » 1 part nettle leaf

To make the tonic:
Prepare an infusion of the herbs, following the instructions on page 29.

To use:
Drink 2 to 3 cups daily.

Mullein

/ Verbascum thapsus

Mullein is certainly one of the most noticeable of wayside weeds, sending stately flowering stalks several feet into the air. In fact, it looks less like a weed and more like an exotic species. Like many wayside weeds, mullein has a long history of effective use in medicine. I love this plant and am always happy to see it on my country walks, in my garden, and on travels around the world.

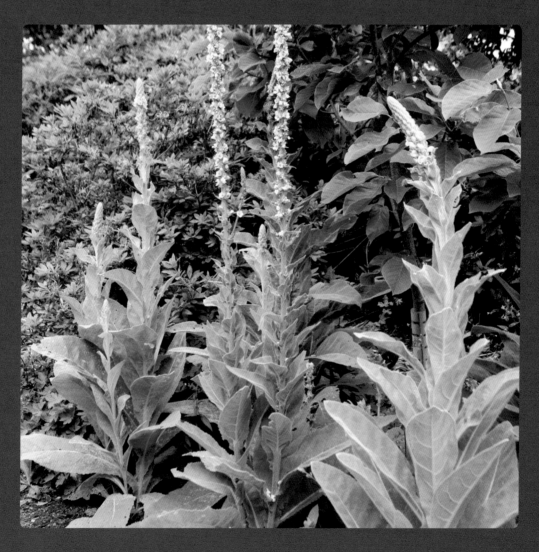

GROWING MULLEIN

Mullein is a biennial; the first year it forms a woolly rosette, and the second year it sends up its tall (up to 7 feet) flowering stalk, sets seed, and then withers and dies. (Leave a few of these mullein stalks standing in the garden; they serve as condominiums for insects, which birds will happily feast on through the long winter months.) Mullein will grow in just about any soil and in any condition. I've seen it growing in woodlands, along railroad tracks, in the meridian of busy freeways, and even in lava fields. But it won't snub its nose at the comfort and luxury of a well-tended garden and will do marvelously planted in full sun in well-drained, nutrient-rich soil with a pH ranging from 5 to 7.5. Mullein is easy to start from seed, and once established in the garden it will self-sow easily. Give it plenty of room to grow and plant it toward the back of a garden or as a centerpiece, as it is has a large and commanding presence. It is very adaptable and will thrive as easily in a Zone 3 garden as one in Zone 8.

MEDICINAL USES

Mullein leaf is both an antispasmodic (it relaxes spasms) and an expectorant (it helps expel mucus), and with these properties it is renowned as a remedy for deep-seated or spastic coughs, bronchial congestion, chest colds, allergies, and other ailments that involve respiratory stress. The leaf can be rolled and smoked with other healing herbs as a treatment for

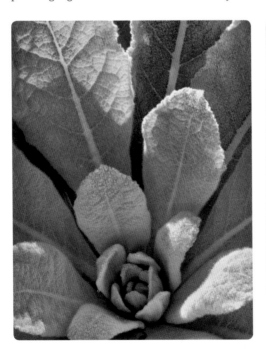

Mullein's large, soft, downy leaves grow from a center rosette.

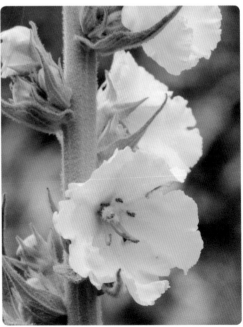

These mullein flowers are ready to harvest.

asthma. The leaf is also a favorite remedy for glandular imbalances, and it's often combined with echinacea root and cleavers in tonics for glandular health. Mullein leaf also makes an effective poultice for boils, glandular swelling, bruises, and insect bites, and it can be added to the bath for relieving rheumatic pain.

The small yellow flowers that creep up the stalk, slowly opening to the sun, are effective anodynes (they relieve pain) with antiseptic and infection-fighting properties. Mullein flower oil has long been famous as an effective treatment for ear infection caused by upper respiratory congestion. Just a few drops of warm oil down each ear will relieve the pain in minutes and reverse the infection in a few days.

Parts used

Leaf, flower, and root

Key constituents

Polysaccharides, flavonoids, sterols, mucilage, saponins

Safety factor

When used externally, the tiny hairs on the underside of the leaves can be irritating to sensitive skin, in which case simply wrap the leaf in cheesecloth or muslin before applying.

Mullein-Red Clover Salve

Apply this salve topically to treat glandular congestion and swelling.

» 1 part calendula flowers
» 1 part mullein leaf
» 1 part red clover flower and leaf
» ½ part mullein flower
» Olive oil
» Grated beeswax

To make the salve:
Infuse the herbs in oil, following the instructions on page 35. Add the beeswax to the oil, following the instructions on page 38, to turn it into a salve.

To use:
Apply a small dab directly to the swollen glands and gently massage into the area.

Mullein Flower Ear Oil

For a "moderate" ear infection caused by the onset of a cold, flu, or other type of upper respiratory congestion, mullein flower oil is the remedy of choice and is amazingly effective not only for fighting the infection but for reducing the pain as well. Of course, if the ear infection doesn't improve with the mullein flower oil treatment within 24 hours, or if it gets worse, a trip to your family health-care provider is in order.

To make the oil:
Collect approximately ¼ cup of mullein flowers just as they open on the flower stalk. It may take a few days to gather a sufficient number of flowers to make the oil, as mullein flowers slowly over several days. Place the flowers in a pint jar and cover with olive oil.

Set the jar in a warm, sunny spot and let infuse for 2 weeks. Strain and bottle. Or make double-strength mullein flower oil: Replace the spent flowers with fresh flowers and let infuse for another 2 weeks. This will make an even more effective remedy.

To use:
Warm the mullein flower oil over very low heat, until it's the temperature of, say, mother's milk. Be sure the oil is *warm*, not hot. If in doubt, do a test drop in your own ear. Dispense 2 or 3 eyedropperfuls of the warm oil down each ear. The ear canals are connected and the infection can move back and forth, so always treat both ears. Repeat two or three times daily, or as often as needed.

Note: *This oil is not effective for "swimmer's ear" and other infections caused by water entering the ear; it will actually make these types of infection worse. And it is not recommended for severe infection, when there's the possibility of eardrum perforation.*

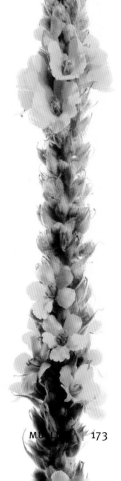

Cough-Be-Gone Tea

A great remedy for coughs and other irritations of the respiratory system.

- » 1 part coltsfoot leaf
- » 1 part marsh mallow leaf and flower
- » 1 part mullein leaf

To make the tea:
Prepare an infusion of the herbs, following the instructions on page 29.

To use:
Drink ½ cup as often as needed until the cough subsides.

Glandular Tonic

The herbs in this blend are particularly beneficial for the entire endocrine gland system.

- » 2 parts mullein flower and leaf
- » 2 parts peppermint or spearmint leaf
- » 1 part calendula flower
- » 1 part cleavers top
- » 1 part red clover flower

To make the tonic:
Prepare this formula as either an infused tea (see page 29) or a tincture (see page 40).

To use:
Drink ½ cup of tea daily, or take ¼ to ½ teaspoon of tincture two or three times daily. Continue for 5 days, discontinue for 2 days, then repeat the cycle as needed.

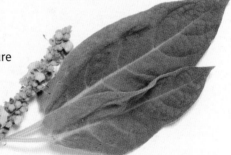

Nettle / *Urtica dioica, U. urens*

With regard to nettle, well-known herbalist Richo Cech sums things up simply in his excellent book *Making Plant Medicine*: "Practical Uses: Legion." Besides the plant's many medicinal uses — including remedies for gout, rheumatism, anemia, exhaustion, menstrual difficulties, skin problems, and hay fever, to mention just a few — nettle can also be cooked and eaten, brewed as beer, infused as tea or tincture, and more. It was once one of the most important plants used in the manufacture of cloth, and many judged nettle fabric to be finer than cotton or linen.

The ancient Greeks and Romans cultivated more acres of nettle than any other crop, and they used it extensively as food and medicine as well as in clothing. Perhaps one of the more unusual uses of nettle

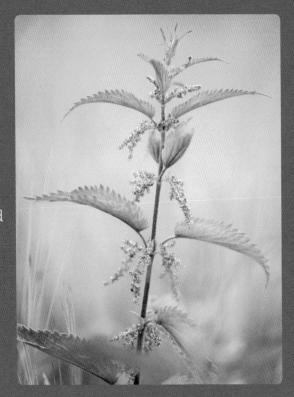

arose out of an old Roman practice called urtication, in which stalks of nettle were cut, tied together, and used to flog arthritic or swollen joints. The resulting nettle rash was reported to improve circulation to the area, thereby relieving aches and pains. Lest you think this treatment antiquated or barbaric, urtication is still in use. And while I'm the first to admit it's not for everyone, it can be as effective as several modern drug treatments for arthritic pain, without the concurrent list of side effects.

And speaking of side effects, I recall a lecture by David Hoffmann, an eminent medical herbalist, at the sixth International Herb Symposium in Boston. After a fascinating 2-hour discourse on the contra-indications and possible side effects of using medicinal plants in conjunction with allopathic medication, Hoffmann concluded with the sweeping statement, "When in doubt, use nettle." Incredibly benevolent (except for its sting) and incredibly beneficial — that's nettle in a nutshell.

GROWING NETTLE

Nettle grows wild throughout the United States and Canada and is easily propagated from runners, which you can gather in the spring or fall from an established stand of plants. The plants prefer fertile, rich soil and the semishaded, moist environments of stream banks. Mimic these conditions in the garden, and nettle will thrive. Also, remember that nettles bite; plant them where you'll not easily brush up against them and where they have room to wander. (You will need to contain them, as they spread rapidly.)

Warning: The herb can and does give a nasty sting. The sting comes from needle-like protrusions on the stems and undersides of the leaves that contain formic acid, the same chemical that causes the pain in bee stings and ant bites. The formic acid is destroyed by heating, drying, or mashing the leaves. Be careful when handling fresh nettle. Wear gloves to harvest it. (Though I must admit, I do know those who harvest it with bare hands to reap the urtification benefits. But be prepared to get stung!)

MEDICINAL USES

Rich in a full spectrum of vitamins and minerals, especially iron and calcium, nettle is an excellent tonic herb and is useful for "growing pains" in young children, when their bones and joints ache, as well as for older folks with "creaky" joints. Its antihistamine properties make it an excellent remedy for allergies and hay fever. Because of its nutritive properties and positive effects on the liver, nettle is also an excellent tonic for the reproductive system of both men and women. It is frequently included in formulas for PMS and other menstrual difficulties, fertility issues, and menopausal issues, and nettle seeds are used as both a preventive and a curative for prostate issues. And I use nettle personally

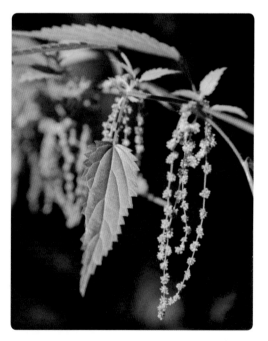

Harvest the nettle leaves before the plant reaches this stage of blossoming.

as a general tonic tea to fortify and build my energy when I'm overworked and tired. This is one of my favorite all-around remedies. In spite or because of its nasty sting, which adds an interesting complexity to its nature, I love this plant.

Best of all, nettle makes it easy to enjoy your medicine. It makes a wonderfully nourishing tea, and in my humble and herb-tainted opinion, there's really no more delicious green than freshly steamed nettles. Pick the nettle tops while still young, using gloves to protect your hands. Steam thoroughly, being certain there are no little stingers left unsteamed. Sprinkle generously with olive oil and fresh lemon juice; serve with a bit of crumbled feta cheese.

Parts used

Primarily the leaf, but also the root (as a tonic for the prostate) and seed (as a general tonic and for increasing stamina and energy)

Key constituents

Calcium, iron, protein, potassium, formic acid, acetylcholine, sulfur, beta-carotene, vitamin K, flavonoids

Safety factor

Despite its "sting," which can most definitely leave large, sore welts, nettle is generally consided a wonderfully safe, edible medicinal plant.

Prostate Tonic Tincture

All men over the age of 50 would be wise to use tonic herbs and foods to nourish and protect their prostate gland. Nettle, especially the root and seed, is a well-known prostate tonic. Take a daily dose along with a handful of pumpkin seeds as an excellent preventive health measure.

» 2 parts nettle root
» 1 part nettle leaf

» 1 part nettle seed
» 80-proof alcohol

To make a tincture:
Tincture the herbs in the alcohol, following the instructions on page 40.

To use:
As a preventive, supporting good health for the prostate, take ½ to 1 teaspoon two or three times daily for 3 months. Discontinue use for 2 to 3 weeks, then repeat the cycle. For greater benefit, add 1 part saw palmetto berries.

Creaky Bones & Achy Joints High-Calcium Tea

A high-calcium tea, this formula is great for young people going through growth spurts as well as for older people with achy joints.

» 2 parts nettle leaf
» 1 part green oat top (milky top of just-ripening oats)
» ½ part horsetail leaf
» A pinch of stevia (optional)

To make the tea:
Prepare the herbs as an infusion, following the instructions on page 29. Sweeten with stevia, if desired.

To use:
Drink 2 to 4 cups of tea per day for 3 to 4 weeks.

Nettle Pesto

There are as many recipes for making pesto as there are cooks in Italy! Here's another to add to the collection.

» 1–2 cups olive oil
» ½ cup chopped pine nuts, walnuts, or cashews
» 2–3 cloves garlic
» Several handfuls freshly picked nettles
» ¼ cup grated Parmesan cheese

To make the pesto:
Combine the olive oil, nuts, and garlic in a blender or food processor and blend until creamy. Add the nettles (yes, raw and unsteamed!) a handful at a time and blend thoroughly, until the pesto becomes a creamy paste. (As long as you blend well, making sure the nettle has been puréed thoroughly, there won't be any sting.) Add the Parmesan and stir well.

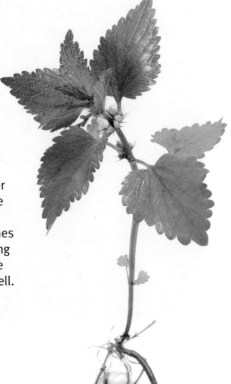

Creamy Nettle-Potato Soup

A perfect "remedy" for those recovering from illness, where a nourishing, easy-to-digest meal is just what the herbalist ordered.

» 1 tablespoon olive oil

» 1 large yellow onion, chopped

» 2–3 medium potatoes, chopped into small cubes

» 2 quarts broth (herbal, vegetable, or chicken)

» Several large handfuls nettle leaf

» Grated Parmesan cheese

» Salt and freshly ground black pepper

To make the soup:
Warm the oil in a large soup pot over medium heat. Add the onion and sauté until soft and golden, about 10 minutes. Add the potatoes and sauté until soft, 8 to 10 minutes.

Add the broth, bring to a boil, then reduce the heat and let simmer until the potatoes are almost tender, about 10 minutes. Then add several large handfuls of fresh nettles to the pot. Cover and let steam until the nettles and potatoes are cooked through, 15 to 20 minutes.

Purée the soup. Season to taste with the Parmesan, salt, and pepper.

Pregnancy Tonic Tea

A delicious, nourishing tea to drink throughout pregnancy, with several essential vitamins and minerals.

» 1 part green oat top (milky top of just-ripening oats)

» 1 part lemon balm leaf

» 1 part nettle leaf

» 1 part raspberry leaf

To make the tonic:
Prepare an infusion of the herbs, following the instructions on page 29.

To use:
Drink 2 to 4 cups daily, or as often as desired, throughout pregnancy.

Oats / *Avena sativa, A. fatua*

Growing up in rural northern California, I was familiar with the nourishing properties of oats. Each fall big flatbed trucks would arrive at our small dairy farm with bales of oatstraw, which our herd of willing bovines eagerly processed into delicious, creamy milk. Later, when I opened my first herb shop and started selling oats for medicinal purposes, my father would joke with me that he was in the wrong business. He may have been right; he was buying oats for $6 a bale to feed the cows, and I was selling it for 50 cents an ounce to help people!

Oats, among the earliest grains to be cultivated, have long been valued as a nutritious cereal for people and farm animals alike and esteemed for their tonic effects. Most herbalists prefer the milky green tops for medicinal purposes, but the oatstraw (the stalk) contains silica as well as other minerals needed for strong bones, hair, teeth, and nails. The milky green tops are especially renowned for their demulcent (soothing) and nourishing effect on the nervous system. The fully ripe oats, often served as heart-healthy oatmeal or ground into oat flour, are also soothing and nourishing.

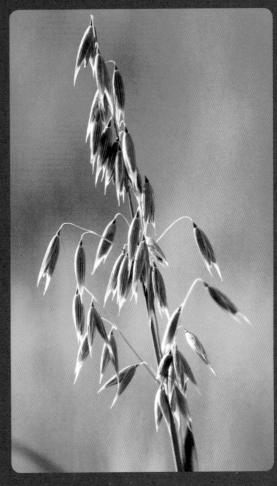

GROWING OATS

We don't normally think of growing oats in the backyard, but why not? These lovely, willowy grains are quite beautiful, their golden stalks bending and swaying in the wind.

Oats are hardy annuals that prefer full sun in open ground. They grow best in Zones 4 through 9 but are adaptable. The seeds germinate readily. Presoak them overnight, then direct-sow into the soil. Keep the soil moist until the seeds have germinated, then water moderately.

For medicinal purposes, oats are ready to harvest when the grains are fully mature but still in their "green" stage — when you press the grain, it should release a tiny bit of "oat milk." For culinary purposes (oatmeal), wait to harvest until the grains are golden and fully ripened. Collect the oats on a sunny morning. Hold a basket in one hand, and use your other hand as a rake, pulling upward, letting the grains fall gracefully into the basket. This peaceful, reflective work is itself "medicine for the nerves" and one of my favorite pastimes.

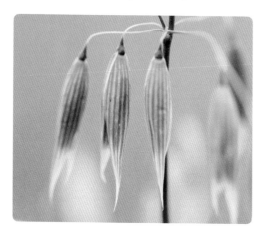

These oats are ready for harvest, green and releasing "oat milk" when gently pinched.

MEDICINAL USES

These days everyone is familiar with the heart-healthy, nutritive properties of oatmeal. But as healthy as oats may be for us, it's the green milky tops that herbalists prefer. Why? The green milky tops of oats make simply one of the best nutritive tonics for the nervous system, effectively relieving all manner of nervous stress, exhaustion, irritation, and anxiety. They are particularly valuable for situations, as in multiple sclerosis, in which the mycelium sheath surrounding nerve endings has been damaged or worn. Though milky oats may not heal multiple sclerosis, they generally lesson the disease's symptoms by reducing fatigue, strengthening the muscles, and improving nerve function.

Milky oats can also be used (particularly in combination with lemon balm) to counteract hyperactivity in children and adults. Combined with damiana root and nettle root, they're used as a sexual tonic for men with impotency problems. And combined with oatstraw (the stalks of the oats), they're often used in formulas to strengthen and heal bones and as a source of dietary calcium, especially during pregnancy and menopause.

Oatmeal, made from the ripe grains, is also healing and is one of those reliable "kitchen medicines" readily available in times of need. For those in convalescence (especially after surgery or during chemotherapy treatments), when nothing else will stay down, a bowl of warm oatmeal porridge is not only nourishing but also soothing and healing, with anti-inflammatory properties. Other nourishing tonic herbs can be added to the porridge for added benefits (see the recipe on page 183).

Oats are also a wonderful topical remedy for soothing skin irritation and itchiness. A warm oatmeal bath is a well-known remedy for irritated, chapped, dry skin. Oatmeal also makes a soothing lotion for sunburn and can be used as a healing facial; simply apply the "milk" from the top of the oatmeal bowl and let it sit on your face for 20 to 30 minutes.

Parts used

Green milky top primarily, though the stalk (oatstraw) and dried oats (oatmeal) are also beneficial

Key constituents

Silicon, sterols, flavonoids, starch, protein, calcium, silica, B vitamins

Safety factor

Oats are perfectly and wonderfully safe (unless you have an allergy).

Oatmeal Bath for Dry, Chapped Skin

Oatmeal baths are a time-honored solution for dry, chapped skin. They're soothing and relaxing for babies, and for the elderly as well.

To prepare the bath:
Make a large pot of runny oatmeal or "oatmeal tea" using four to six times more water than oats. Cook for 15 minutes, then strain, reserving both the liquid and the oats. Fill a bathtub with warm water, then add the cooking liquid directly to the bathtub. Scoop the cooked oats into a muslin bag, nylon stocking, or large cotton cloth and tie tightly closed. For added benefit, add a drop or two of lavender essential oil to the bath to enhance the relaxing effects.

To use:
Get in and enjoy the relaxing, soothing effects. Use the oats bag as a gentle scrub by massaging it over your skin.

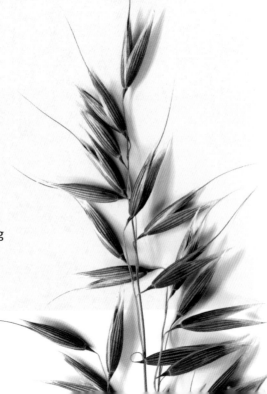

Heart-Healthy Oatmeal

Be creative with oatmeal; it's a great medium to mix many herbs into!

To make the oatmeal:
Make a bowl of oatmeal following the directions on the container. To each cup of cooked oatmeal, add 2 teaspoons hawthorn berry powder. Stir in dried elderberries, fresh or dried goji berries, and/or fresh or dried blueberries for added antioxidant benefits. Flavor with a dab of honey or maple syrup and a sprinkle of cinnamon.

To use:
Enjoy as a healthy start to a new day.

Restorative Oatmeal Porridge

Oatmeal porridge is an easy-to-digest, nourishing food and the addition of medicinal herbs makes it a healing meal. Feel free to add other herbs for addressing a particular illness.

>> 1 teaspoon green oat top (milky top of just-ripening oats)

>> 1 teaspoon chopped hawthorn berry

>> 1 teaspoon chopped Siberian ginseng root

>> ½ cup oatmeal

>> ½ teaspoon hawthorn berry powder

>> ½ teaspoon rhodiola root powder

>> ½ teaspoon Siberian ginseng root powder

>> Maple syrup, honey, cinnamon, and/or miso (optional)

To make the porridge:
Combine the green oat tops, chopped hawthorn berry, and chopped Siberian ginseng with 2 cups of water in a saucepan. Bring to a boil, then remove from the heat, cover, and let sit for 30 to 45 minutes. Strain, composting the spent herbs. Add the oatmeal to the tea. Bring to a boil, then reduce the heat and let simmer until the oats are cooked, 10 to 15 minutes. The porridge will be runnier than regular oatmeal. Add the powdered hawthorn, rhodiola, and Siberian ginseng and mix well. Flavor with maple syrup, honey, and/or cinnamon, or use miso for a heartier soup flavor.

Peppermint is often referred to as "a blast of green energy." It renews, refreshes, and energizes without depleting or using up energy reserves. When you need a gentle pick-me-up, try peppermint and holy basil tea, which will gently restore and revitalize. Or try peppermint in a "brain tonic," combined with ginkgo, gotu kola, and rosemary, where it will help bolster your memory and sharpen your thinking. Few herbs are as versatile, delicious, safe, effective, readily available, and easy to grow as peppermint.

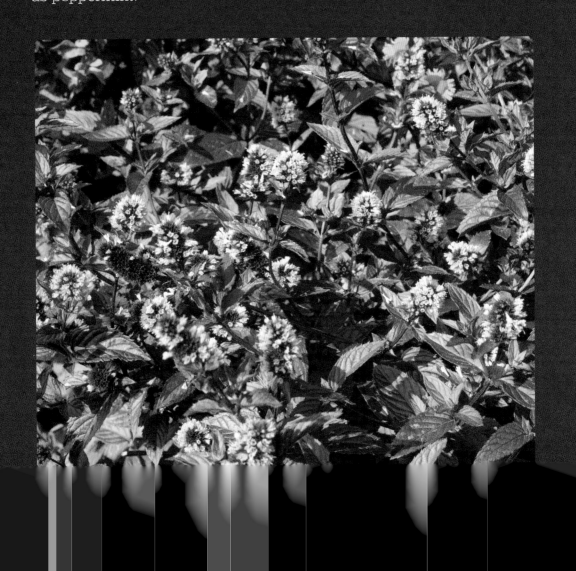

GROWING PEPPERMINT

Peppermint prefers rich, moist, well-drained soil and full sun to partial shade. It does best in Zones 5 through 9, but don't be afraid to experiment if you live in a colder zone, because peppermint, like most mints, has a wild spirit and is a survivor.

Peppermint starts easily from root divisions and cuttings. In fact, the most challenging aspect of growing peppermint, or any other mint, is keeping it contained. You might consider growing peppermint in a container to keep it from taking over the garden. Of course, the best way to keep peppermint from spreading beyond its place in the garden is to continue to harvest it for teas, cooking, herbal remedies, and mint juleps!

MEDICINAL USES

Peppermint is renowned as a digestive aid and is the herb of choice for relieving nausea and gas. As an antispasmodic, it helps muscles relax and can reduce stomach cramping and spasms, and its clean, refreshing flavor is welcome after a bout of indigestion or vomiting. A drop or two of peppermint essential oil in a cup of warm water quickly removes the foul taste and odor left after stomach upset. It's a common ingredient in toothpastes, mouthwashes, and chewing gum. In fact, peppermint is probably the flavor that defines fresh breath and a clean mouth. Even cleaning products are prone to include peppermint for the clean, fresh scent it imparts. Use it as a disinfectant spray in the bathroom; everything seems to perk up.

Not so well known are peppermint's anodyne properties. It's one of my favorite herbs for reducing the pain of headaches, bee stings, burns, and even toothache. For burns, add a drop or two of peppermint essential oil to 2 tablespoons of honey and apply directly to the burn. Honey makes an excellent sterile dressing for the burn, while the peppermint cools and relieves the pain, usually within minutes. And peppermint tea can help reduce the pain and duration of a headache, especially one caused by a digestive problem. Try tea made with equal parts of chamomile and peppermint for indigestion and headaches caused by indigestion.

Because of its delicious and familiar flavor, peppermint is often used in conjunction with other, less tasty medicinal herbs. And it contains an assortment of important nutrients, including calcium, magnesium, and potassium. Add it to blender drinks, soups, salads, and pestos for its refreshing flavor and nutritional value.

Parts used

Leaf and flower

Key constituents

Volatile oils (menthol and menthone), flavonoids, phenolic acid, triterpines, calcium, magnesium, potassium

Safety factor

Perfectly safe; no known reactions or harmful side effects

PEPPERMINT

Rejuvenation Tonic

A lightly uplifting tea, perfect for a morning wake-up or an afternoon pick-me-up.

» 1 part green tea (optional)
» 1 part holy basil leaf
» 1 part peppermint leaf

To make the tonic:
Prepare the herbs as an infusion, following the instructions on page 29.

To use:
Drink 1 cup as needed throughout the day. Because of the caffeine in green tea, avoid drinking this tonic in the evening, as it might interfere with sleep.

Headache Tincture

This remedy is especially helpful for those who are prone to headaches that stem from indigestion.

» 2 parts peppermint leaf
» 1 part chamomile flower
» 1 part feverfew flower and leaf
» 1 part hops strobile
» 80-proof alcohol

To make the tincture:
Tincture the herbs in the alcohol, following the instructions on page 40.

To use:
Take ¼ to ½ teaspoon before and after meals.

MINT SEGREGATION

Mints intermingle and "interbreed" quite readily, so if you grow more than one type, you can end up with all manner of mints, most of which won't taste or smell as nice as the parent plants. They won't be as medicinally active either. So attempt to keep your mints separated, or at least in different beds or pots in the garden; they are not good bedmates.

Digestive Aid

This simple tea is probably one of the most well-known herbal formulas for upset tummies and indigestion.

» 1 part chamomile flower
» 1 part dill leaf and seed
» 1 part peppermint leaf

To make the tea:
Prepare the herbs as an infusion, following the instructions on page 29.

To use:
Drink ½ cup of the warm tea before and after meals.

Peppermint Tooth Powder

Did you know you can easily make effective, good-tasting, and inexpensive toothpaste yourself? And it's even easy! You can actually find tubes for your homemade toothpaste at cosmetics and camping stores.

» ¼ cup finely powdered Kaolin clay
» 1 teaspoon baking soda
» 1 teaspoon finely ground sea salt
» A few drops of peppermint essential oil

To make the powder:
Combine the powdered clay, baking soda, salt, and essential oil and mix well. Allow to air-dry, then store in an airtight container.

To use:
Mix the tooth powder with enough peppermint tea or water to make a moist paste. (If you make the powder in large batches, moisten only enough for a week or two at a time, so the toothpaste doesn't spoil.) If you like the sweet taste of most toothpastes — I don't — add a teaspoon of vegetable glycercin to the paste. Use to brush your teeth, like store-bought toothpaste.

Plantain / *Plantago major, P. lanceolata*

I suspect plantain takes second place, just behind dandelion, in the category of "most common and most useful weed." It grows everywhere: in lawns and empty lots, in cracks in sidewalks, on highways and pathways, on the beach, in meadows, in backyards, and in wild places. Few plants we tend in our gardens are as dependable or as useful as plantain.

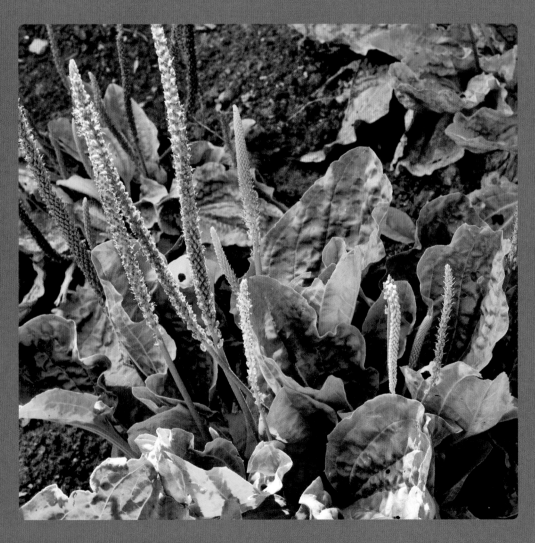

GROWING PLANTAIN

I'm trying to imagine why anyone would want to cultivate plantain, when it's most certainly already growing somewhere in your neighborhood — perhaps even in your own backyard or your vegetable garden. If you don't have a ready stock of plantain already growing, just till up a little soil — preferably in full sun — water it infrequently, and wait: Plantain will show up! It always accepts an invitation to join you in your garden. If you get impatient, collect some ripe seeds from your neighbor's patch and sprinkle them in your freshly tilled soil. Next year you'll have your own private patch of this "super herb" and be the envy of the neighborhood.

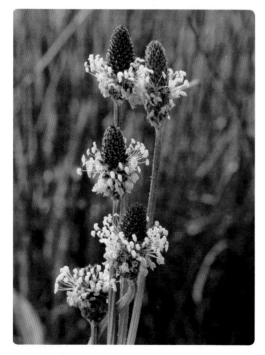

Though considered a lowly weed, common plantain is quite lovely when it flowers.

MEDICINAL USES

Plantain draws toxicity from the body. It has a long history of use as a remedy for blood poisoning and is considered an "alterative" (blood purifier) in the old sense of the word; its rich nutrients stimulate the liver and enrich or "cleanse" the blood. It is used for all manner of liver problems, including poor digestion and assimilation, hepatitis, jaundice, skin eruptions, and eruptive personalities (too much heat in the body).

Plantain is the poultice herb supreme. The leaves can be chopped, mashed, and placed directly over the problem area. Or they can be made into a strong tea, and a cloth soaked in the tea is placed directly over the area. As a poultice, plantain is a highly effective remedy for the bites and stings of insects, boils and other eruptive skin disorders, and any deep-seated infection. Plantain has such excellent drawing properties that it can be used to remove slivers that are too deep to pull out. Soak the area of the sliver in a very hot plantain tea for 20 to 30 minutes. You can increase the effectiveness of the tea by adding a tablespoon or two of sea salt. Then apply mashed plantain leaves and wrap in place. Change the poultice two or three times during the day if possible, and repeat this cycle until the sliver is close enough to the surface of the skin to pull out.

Plantain also has styptic and hemostatic properties, meaning that it can help check bleeding. Place the mashed herbs directly on the wound until the blood flow slows or stops. As a tea or tincture, plantain can also be used to stanch heavy menstrual bleeding. Though it can be used alone to stop bleeding, it's more effective when blended with yarrow and nettle (or shepherd's purse) for this purpose. It's also an excellent wound healer and shortens recovery time.

Plantain is nutrient dense, containing protein, starch, and a host of vitamins, and is an excellent emergency food. Though it can be bitter and stringy as it gets older, it's a tasty ingredient in many wild-food dishes.

The plantain seeds, which grow at the top of a long slender stalk, are rich in mucilage and mildly laxative. A cultivated variety of plantain, *P. psyllium*, is grown for its large, abundant seeds, which are used as bulk laxatives. Psyllium seed is the main ingredient in Metamucil.

For anything to be this common, nutritious, safe, and effective, not to mention free for the picking, is truly a gift to humankind. If plantain put on a fancy name, donned an exotic blossom, and hailed from anywhere other than our own backyards and empty fields, we'd call it a super food, extol its virtues, and put a hefty price tag on it.

Parts used
Seed, root, and leaf

Key constituents
Mucilage, fatty acids, protein, starch, B vitamins, vitamin C, vitamin K, allantoin, bitters

Safety factor
Perfectly safe; no known reactions or harmful side effects

Plantain Poultice

Poultices are used to draw infection or foreign objects (such as slivers) from the body. Many herbs are used in poultices, but plantain is the most well known, the best of the best.

To make the poultice:
Gather fresh young plantain leaves and mash or chop them.

To use:
Place the mashed herbs directly against the skin, then wrap a cloth over them to hold them in place. Or, if you prefer, wrap the herbs in a thin cloth and place the cloth against the skin. Leave on for 30 to 45 minutes, changing the wrap as necessary. The herbs may turn black and become very hot, which is a sign that toxins are being drawn out. Discard the herbs and reapply a new poultice.

Plantain Power Drink

Green drinks have become quite popular — and quite expensive! So why not use the nourishing greens that grow wild in your garden and backyard, free for the picking? Packed with nutrition, this power drink is also packed with goodness.

» 2–3 cups fresh or canned (unsweetened) pineapple juice

» A handful of plantain leaves (and/or other nutritive herbs, such as red clover flower, raspberry leaf, self-heal flower and leaf, and mint leaf)

» 1 banana, peeled

To make the drink:
Combine all the ingredients in a blender and blend thoroughly. Adjust flavor to taste.

To use:
Drink a cup of this nutritive tonic each day.

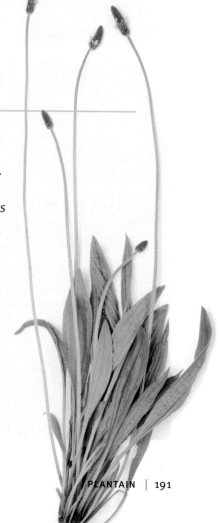

Plantain Salve

Plantain salve is the ultimate "boo-boo" salve, good for just about any kind of skin infection or irritation. Making plantain salve is a great project to do with kids. You can get creative with the recipe, adding different herb combinations or essential oils. Other good choices are yarrow, red clover, burdock leaf, self-heal (Prunella vulgaris), mint . . . the possibilities are endless.

To make the salve:
Make a salve of plantain leaf, following the instructions on page 38.

To use:
Apply a small dab directly to the affected area. Repeat a few times throughout the day until the problem has subsided.

Red Clover / *Trifolium pratense*

Red clover has a highly eclectic fan club. Farmers use it as an inexpensive, quick-growing food for livestock and as a nitrogen-fixing ground cover. Cows love it. Bees gorge on it and go on to make the world's most popular honey. Environmentalists appreciate it because it helps prevent roadside erosion. Gardeners enjoy it as a lovely ground cover. And for herbalists, it's been long valued as a reliable and effective medicine.

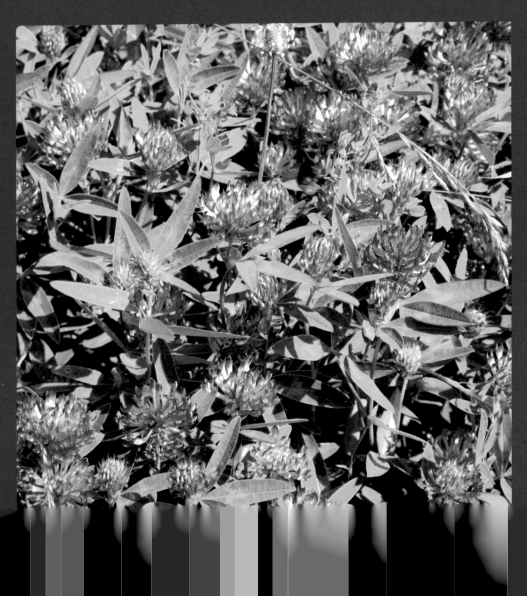

GROWING RED CLOVER

A hardy perennial, red clover is easy to sow and quick to grow. It does well in Zones 4 through 9 and prefers loamy, well-drained soil and full sun. However, like most of the herbs profiled in this book, red clover isn't fussy and will settle for a wide variety of growing situations. It's a legume, and like all members of the Leguminosae family, red clover sends roots deep into the earth and fixes nitrogen in the soil. Though generally considered a plant for fields and meadows, red clover is actually lovely in the garden and provides nectar for honeybees and other pollinating insects. It can be planted in small clumps among other low-growing herbs or given a small plot in the lawn, where it will make itself quite at home. (Were you to let your lawn grow for 2 to 3 weeks, you'd find that all manner of wild medicinal plants were there all along!)

Red clover's pretty pink blossoms bloom throughout the summer and can be harvested just as soon as they open. Use fresh or dry. I like walking through the garden "grazing" as I go, and red clover is always such a delectable treat.

MEDICINAL USES

Red clover offers a rich bounty of nutrients that support the entire body. High in beta-carotene, calcium, vitamin C, a whole spectrum of B vitamins, and essential trace minerals such as magnesium, manganese, zinc, copper, and selenium, this little wildflower truly can be considered one of nature's best vitamin and mineral supplements.

Red clover has a long history of use as a blood and lymphatic cleanser. It is often included in formulas for skin problems such as eczema and psoriasis, whether taken internally or used externally as a wash, and it's a favorite herb for treating lymphatic congestion. It remains my favorite herb for treating childhood respiratory problems and effectively restores vitality and health following a respiratory infection.

Red clover is also a favorite herb for many menopausal women. Both the flowers and leaves contain phytoestrogens (plant hormones) and isoflavones that have a beneficial effect on menopausal symptoms such as hot flashes, mood swings, and night sweats. There's even some recent evidence to indicate red clover might be helpful in maintaining healthy bone density. An excellent blend for menopausal symptoms such as hot flashes and mood swings is red clover, sage, and motherwort. Though the role of isoflavones in the body is not completely understood, they appear to bind with estrogen receptor sites, preventing less healthy forms of estrogen such as estradiol and/or excess estrogen from accumulating. Excess estrogen in the system is believed to be one of the causes of cancer and some menopausal disorders.

Though the U.S. Food and Drug Administration dismisses red clover completely, stating that "there is not sufficient reason to suspect it of any medicinal value," studies conducted by the National Cancer Institute determined that red clover has at least four important antitumor compounds. It's certainly not a cure for cancer, but there's enough evidence to suggest that red clover should be considered, at least, as a preventive agent and perhaps incorporated in a health-promoting tea for those who might be susceptible to cancer.

All this and it's delicious, too . . . as any honeybee will demonstrate! Red clover makes a superlative tonic tea, delicious by itself or with peppermint, spearmint, violet leaf, and other invigorating herbs (see the recipe on page 195). It's a marvelous food, too. The fresh blossoms taste like little honey cups, and I often add them to salads, blender drinks, and garden-fresh soups.

Though the leaves are used medicinally, it is the blossoms of the clover that are prized. They are at their prime when a bright pink or red. Don't harvest flowers that are turning brown, and when buying dried herbs, be wary of brownish blossoms.

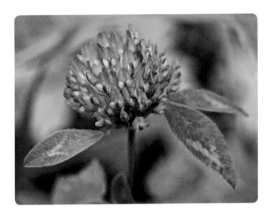

Tasty and gourmet, red clover blossoms are adored by bees, birds, animals, and herbalists!

Parts used

Flowering top and leaf (although the leaf is not as potent)

Key constituents

Polysaccharides, isoflavones, salicylates, coumarins, cyanogenic glycosides, protein, beta-carotene, B vitamins, vitamin C, iron, silicon

Safety factor

Red clover has blood-thinning properties and should not be used by those who are taking heart medication or who have any type of blood-thinning problem. Discontinue red clover for 2 weeks before and after surgery.

Red Clover Vitamin Tonic

This tea comprises some of our common "super-food" herbs, which all contain high concentrations of vitamins and minerals.

» 3 parts red clover flower and leaf

» 2 parts green oat top (milky top of just-ripening oats)

» 2 parts peppermint or spearmint leaf

» 1 part nettle leaf

» 1 part violet leaf

» Honey (optional)

To make the tonic:
Prepare an infusion of the herbs, following the instructions on page 29, and letting them steep for 15 to 20 minutes. Sweeten with honey if desired.

To use:
Drink 2 to 3 cups daily.

Menopause Formula

This lovely formula helps regulate hot flashes and eases some of the discomfort of menopause. Try it and see if you don't notice a difference.

» 2 parts red clover flower

» 1 part lemon balm top

» 1 part motherwort leaf

» 1 part sage leaf

To make the formula:
Prepare the herbs as an infusion, following the instructions on page 29, or as a tincture, following the instructions on page 40.

To use:
Drink 3 or 4 cups of tea a day, or take ¼ to ½ teaspoon of tincture a day for 5 or 6 days. Discontinue for a couple of days, then repeat the cycle as needed.

Flower Power Formula for Lymphatic Congestion

If you tend toward swollen glands or a fibrocystic breast condition, or you have had cancer in the past, this is a good formula to use fairly consistently.

» 2 parts red clover flower
» 1 part calendula flower
» 1 part violet leaf

To make the formula:
Prepare the herbs as an infusion, following the instructions on page 29, or as a tincture, following the instructions on page 40.

To use:
Drink 2 to 3 cups of tea daily, or take ¼ to ½ teaspoon of tincture daily. Continue for 3 weeks, then discontinue for 2 weeks and repeat as needed.

Red Clover–Violet Syrup

A sweet, delicious remedy for lymphatic congestion.

» 1 part calendula flower
» 1 part red clover flower
» 1 part violet leaf (and flower, if available)

To make the syrup:
Prepare the herbs as a syrup, following the instructions on page 33.

To use:
The trick here is not to overindulge in this lovely, sweet syrup! Take ½ to 1 teaspoon two times daily or as often as needed.

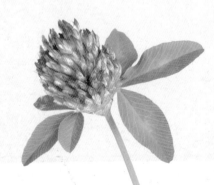

St. John's Wort / *Hypericum perforatum*

St. John's wort has a rich and colorful history. From the time of the ancient Greeks down through the Middle Ages and onward, the herb was considered to be imbued with magical powers and was used to ward off evil and protect against illness. Dioscorides, the famed Greek herbalist, mentioned the use of St. John's wort for sciatica and other nerve problems. Theophrastus recommended it for external wounds and cuts, and both Galen and Paracelsus included it as an important healing herb in their pharmacopoeia. St. John's wort's fame has endured through the ages, and though its uses — and the terminology explaining how it may work — have changed slightly over the centuries, it is still as popular as ever as a valuable medicinal herb.

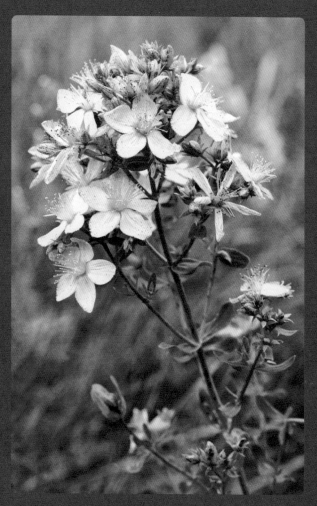

GROWING ST. JOHN'S WORT

Those new to gardening will be encouraged to know that St. John's wort is generally considered a hardy weed and most people try to eradicate it rather than grow it in the garden. It's a sun-loving, hardy perennial, preferring full sun and somewhat dry soil, but it's not fussy and will do almost as well in partial shade and some drenching. It thrives in Zones 3 through 9, and prefers soil with a pH of 6 to 7. It's rather rangy, growing to 3 or 4 feet on long, spare stalks. But when in full bloom St. John's wort is a beauty, lighting up its section of the garden with small sun-flecked flowers. It germinates easily from seed, though seeds need to be stratified (treated to a winterlike chill) for best germination. Once established in your garden, it will readily self-sow. You can purchase a plant or two from an herb nursery (most regular nurseries won't carry St. John's wort) to start off. But make sure you're getting *H. perforatum*. There are several species, some considered more handsome for the garden and therefore more available, but none is as medicinal as the wild *H. perforatum*.

St. John's wort has naturalized in many parts of the globe and can be found growing wild in sunny meadows, on dry hillsides, and even in open fields along roadways. *H. perforatum* is distinctive because of the tiny oil glands in the leaf; when held to the light, they look like tiny pinpricks covering the surface of the leaf.

Gathering St. John's wort is an afternoon pleasure, and one that's been enjoyed through the ages. Always gather on a sunny day, when the flowers will be dry.

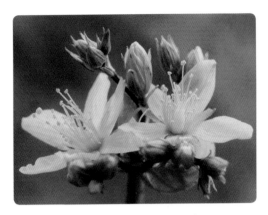

St. John's wort is ready to pick when the buds are full and ready to open.

The flowers are at their best just as the buds begin to open. To tell if they are ready, press a bud between your fingers. If there's a spurt of purple or deep red, the buds are ready. If not, it's either too early or too late. Check daily. The window for optimum harvesting is short.

MEDICINAL USES

St. John's wort can be very effective for treating mild depression, anxiety, stress, tension, nerve damage, and seasonal affective disorder (SAD). About 10 years ago, after its five minutes of fame on *60 Minutes*, in a segment that highlighted St. John's wort's use for depression and anxiety, its popularity shot off the charts; sales were up 400 percent almost overnight. While St. John's wort is potent, it is not a drug, and it does not have druglike instantaneous actions. Like many herbs, it needs to be used over a period of time for full effect. To be effective against stress and depression, St. John's wort needs to be taken over a 2- to 3-week period, and it is often cycled over several months to treat chronic depression and stress. Unfortunately, this wasn't made clear in the newscast, and many of those who raced out to try St. John's wort in place of their antidepressants were disappointed.

However, used correctly and appropriately, St. John's wort is a very effective antidepressant, and over the past 30 years its efficacy has been proved by extensive clinical and scientific studies. Hypericin, one of the herb's active constituents, increases the metabolism of serotonin and melatonin, which aid the body's ability to receive and store light. Hyperforin, another important constituent, contributes to emotional stability by slowing the uptake of those "feel-good" neurotransmitters such as dopamine, serotonin, and noradrenaline, allowing them to circulate longer in the body. This may explain, in part, St. John's wort's ability to "lift the spirits" and relieve depression.

Whether taken internally or applied topically, St. John's wort has marked antibacterial, antiviral, and anti-inflammatory properties, which make it helpful for treating bacterial and viral infections such as shingles and herpes. And there have been some promising studies done on St. John's wort's ability to inhibit the AIDS virus, but research is still ongoing.

The rich red oil made from the bright yellow flowers is simply one of the best remedies for trauma to the skin. It is applied topically to soothe and heal bruises, sprains, burns, and injuries of all kinds. It not only relieves pain but also promotes tissue repair and speeds recovery.

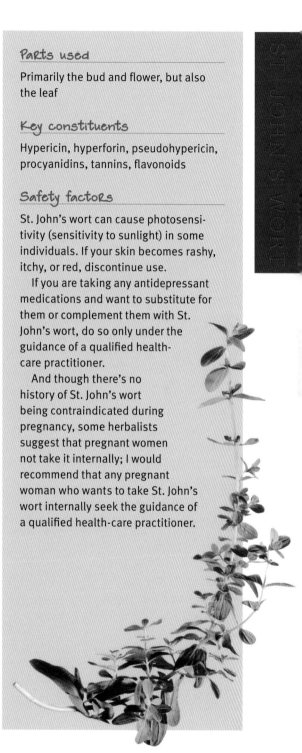

Parts used
Primarily the bud and flower, but also the leaf

Key constituents
Hypericin, hyperforin, pseudohypericin, procyanidins, tannins, flavonoids

Safety factors
St. John's wort can cause photosensitivity (sensitivity to sunlight) in some individuals. If your skin becomes rashy, itchy, or red, discontinue use.

If you are taking any antidepressant medications and want to substitute for them or complement them with St. John's wort, do so only under the guidance of a qualified health-care practitioner.

And though there's no history of St. John's wort being contraindicated during pregnancy, some herbalists suggest that pregnant women not take it internally; I would recommend that any pregnant woman who wants to take St. John's wort internally seek the guidance of a qualified health-care practitioner.

St. John's wort Oil

Perhaps one of the most traditional herbal oils, the colorful red oil made from St. John's wort flowers has been used for centuries as first aid for burns, bruises, and other trauma to the skin. And it's still as popular as ever. Recently, when traveling through Switzerland, I stopped at a little family restaurant for lunch. Lining the windowsills were colorful bottles of St. John's wort oil brewing in the sun.

St. John's wort oil is best made from the buds, with some flowers and leaves (the approximate proportions — and they are only approximate — are 70 percent buds and 30 percent flowers and leaves). Pick the buds when they are fully ripened and just ready to open, and the flowers when they are freshly opened. It's easy to tell when the buds and flowers are at their peak: Pinch them, and if your fingers stain bright red, they are ready. If not, wait. . . . But don't wait too long. If you miss the opportunity, that day or two when the flowers and buds are at their peak, you'll have to wait for a full year before making your St. John's wort oil.

To make the oil:

Place the freshly picked St. John's wort in a glass jar and cover with an inch or two of olive oil. The buds may float for a while, but they should settle down eventually. Place in direct sunlight (a sunny window works well) and let infuse for 2 to 3 weeks. As the herb steeps, the oil will become a deep, almost fluorescent red. The deeper and richer the color, the better the product. When it's ready, strain and bottle.

To use:

Simply spread the oil over the burn, bruise, cut, or other skin injury. It is also helpful for treating ear infections; add some to your garlic oil (see page 77). Because it is useful for healing nerve damage, it can be helpful in cases of Bell's palsy, multiple sclerosis, and other diseases of the nervous system.

variation

Some people prefer to roughly pulse the oil and buds together in a blender; it gives the blend a head start on the maceration process and also eliminates bud float.

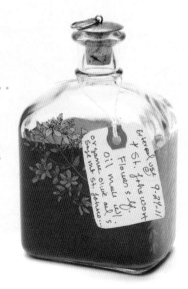

St. John's Wort Salve

An excellent, all-purpose salve for rashes (including diaper rash), burns, cuts, and wounds, I first made it back in 1974 and found it so effective that I have been making it ever since.

» 1 part calendula flower
» 1 part comfrey leaf
» 1 part St. John's wort leaf and flower
» Olive oil
» Beeswax

To make the salve:
Infuse each herb in oil, following the instructions on page 35. Then use the herbal oils (in equal portions) and the beeswax to make a salve, following the instructions on page 38.

To use:
Use a small dab on any wound, cut, burn, or skin injury that needs healing.

St. John's Wort Liniment

This recipe comes courtesy of fellow herbalist Nancy Phillips. It is my favorite liniment and remedy of choice for treating sore muscles, spastic muscles and cramps, and painful joints (including those caused by arthritis and bursitis).

To make the liniment:
There's a two-part process in making this liniment. Make at least 1 pint of St. John's wort tincture, following the instructions on page 40, but using pure grain alcohol (190 proof or higher) instead of 80-proof alcohol. At the same time, make at least 1 pint of of St. John's Wort Oil, following the instructions on page 200.

After 3 to 4 weeks of steeping, when the oil and the tincture are both a deep rich red, strain. Combine 1 pint of tincture with 1 pint of oil and add several drops of wintergreen essential oil. Label and store in a cool place, where the liniment will keep for at least several months.

To use:
Use this liniment any time your muscles, joints, or bones are aching for some attention. It's not only pain relieving but reaches deep into the muscles to relieve spasms and relax tightness as well.

St. John's Wort Lighten-Up Tea

It's said that St. John's wort flowers help "bring light into our lives." For a little light, or lightening up, try this tea.

- » 2 parts St. John's wort flower
- » 1 part green oat top (milky top of just-ripening oats)
- » 1 part lemon balm leaf
- » 1 part spearmint leaf
- » A pinch of stevia

To make the tea:
Prepare an infusion of the herbs (including the stevia), following the instructions on page 29.

To use:
Drink 3 to 4 cups daily, as needed.

St. John's Wort Tincture for SAD (Seasonal Affective Disorder)

Seasonal affective disorder (SAD) is not uncommon in my far-northern corner of the world, where winters are long and dark. Getting outdoors, keeping active, breathing the cold air, and using this tincture all help keep sunshine in our hearts.

- » 2 parts St. John's wort flower
- » 1 part green oat top (milky top of just-ripening oats)
- » 1 part hawthorn leaf, flower, and berry
- » 80-proof alcohol

To make the tincture:
Tincture the herbs in alcohol, following the instructions on page 40.

To use:
Take ½ to 1 teaspoon twice daily for 3 weeks. Discontinue for 1 week, then repeat the cycle as needed. Or, alternatively, take the tincture for 5 days, discontinue for 2 days, then repeat the cycle as needed.

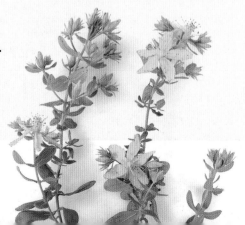

Spearmint / *Mentha spicata*

Cooling, refreshing, and uplifting, spearmint is second only to peppermint as the most popular of all the mints. It's also considered the oldest; most other mints, including peppermint, are offspring of spearmint, her wildly prolific progeny. Though often hiding shyly in the garden behind more colorful plants, and sometimes overlooked in the herbal pantry, spearmint is nonetheless a valuable and tasty addition to the home apothecary.

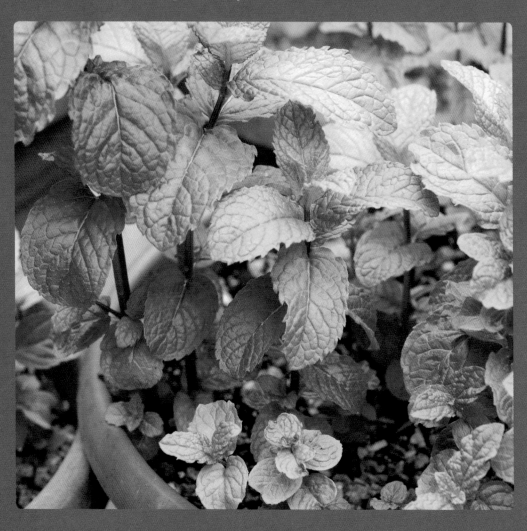

GROWING SPEARMINT

Spearmint is a quick-growing perennial in Zones 4 through 9. Like most mints, it spreads by runners. It's easy to start from root divisions and/or cuttings, but you won't want to start it from seed. As is the case for most mints, the seeds won't be true to type, and often seed-started mints are less potent than the parent plant. Spearmint especially thrives near water. It's lovely planted by a pond; if no pond is available, try planting it in rich soil by a water spigot or gutter downspout, so that it catches the runoff. It's not particularly fussy about soil type, though it does prefer rich, moist soil and partial shade. And if you're growing spearmint with other types of mints, keep them separated (see the box on page 186).

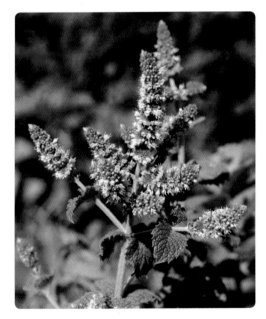

Spearmint is considered the mother of all mints, as it is generally thought to be the oldest of mints.

MEDICINAL USES

Though spearmint is often passed over in favor of its stronger-flavored cousin, peppermint, there are times when I definitely prefer to use spearmint in my herbal blends. Spearmint is sweeter, milder, and less pungent than peppermint and tends to be better for children. Combined with catnip, it's an excellent herb for children with a fever. Or blend it in equal proportions with lemon balm to calm hyperactivity and anxiety in children.

Spearmint is a mild digestive aid and is lovely as a before-dinner aperitif or after-dinner digestif. Simply make a strong tea and mix with sparking water, and perhaps a handful of fresh raspberries or blueberries.

Spearmint is one of those herbs with amphoteric properties; it seems to move in the direction the body needs. It's a mild stimulant but also has relaxing properties, and so it's perfect in blends for strengthening the nervous system, both calming and energizing at the same time. It also has both warming and cooling properties: As the menthol evaporates, it imparts a cooling sensation to the skin and digestive system, but as the herb penetrates, it stimulates blood flow, causing a warm sensation.

Spearmint's well-known refreshing flavor is used in everything from toothpaste and mouthwash to soda and tea. It is delicious in salads, grain dishes, cold soups, fresh fruit compotes, and sliced fruit dishes. You can certainly use the wonderful flavor in an herbal blend to cover up the flavor of other, less tasty herbs. And you can use spearmint to "sweeten" the mouth after sickness; it is especially helpful to get rid of that sour taste that follows vomiting. Just add a drop of the essential oil to water or make a cup of fresh spearmint tea, and use it to rinse out your mouth several times. Spearmint also helps settle a restless stomach and is often combined with ginger for this purpose. It's a wonderful addition to any uplifting, mildly stimulating herbal blend, and it is delicious infused in honey for a quick pick-me-up.

Parts used

Primarily the leaf, but also the flower

Key constituents

Essential oils, B vitamins, vitamin C, potassium, flavonoids, tannins

Safety factor

Generally regarded as safe

Iced Spearmint Tea

I'm not sure that iced spearmint tea would be considered a "medicinal" except in the purest sense; it's a delicious drink that's healthy, makes you feel good, and is packed with nutrition. Mints contain a whole spectrum of vitamins and minerals, including beta-carotene, vitamin C, potassium, flavonoids, menthol, and essential oils.

To make the tea:

Make a double-strong infusion of spearmint leaf, following instructions on page 29 and doubling the amount of herb. Add ice cubes, or chill in the refrigerator. Sweeten with stevia or honey, add a few springs of fresh spearmint and a sliced lemon, and serve. (It's also nice with a handful of fresh berries or mixed with sparkling water.)

To use:

Enjoy. Nothing could be nicer on a hot summer day.

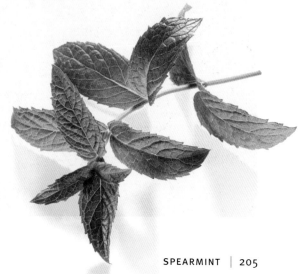

Fever-Reducing Formula for children

This is a time-tested, renowned formula for reducing mild fevers in children. Of course, for any persistent or high fever, consult with your health-care professional.

» 1 part catnip leaf
» 1 part elder flower
» 1 part spearmint leaf
» Stevia (optional)
» Maple syrup (optional)

To make the tea:
Prepare an infusion of the herbs (including the stevia, if using), following the instructions on page 29. Sweeten to taste with maple syrup, if using.

To use:
For children 3 to 6 years of age, give ¼ cup every 2 hours until the fever subsides. For children younger than 3, give 1 teaspoon per year of age.

children's Stress calmer Glycerite

A gentle, calming remedy for children (and adults as well).

» 1 part chamomile flower
» 1 part lemon balm leaf
» 1 part spearmint leaf
» 75% glycerin solution (3 parts glycerin to 1 part water)

To make glycerite:
Tincture the herbs in the glycerin solution, following the instructions on page 40 and letting the herbs steep for 3 to 4 weeks.

To use:
For children 3 to 6 years of age, give ½ teaspoon two or three times daily. For children 6 to 10 years of age, give ¾ to 1 teaspoon two or three times daily. For children younger than 3, adjust the dose according to weight and size (see the chart on page 48).

Evening Repose

A calming, uplifting tea blend, perfect after work or a long, stressful day.

» 2 parts spearmint leaf
» 1 part chamomile flower
» 1 part lemon balm leaf
» ½ part rose petal
» A pinch of stevia to sweeten (optional)

To make the tea:
Prepare an infusion of the herbs (including the stevia), following the instructions on page 29.

To use:
Drink a cup or two in the evening after dinner, sitting in the rocker on your front porch, enjoying the sunset . . .

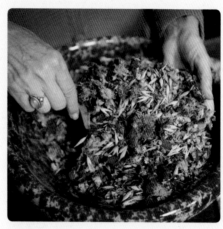

Once you learn to make tea blends, you can develop your own combinations, such as this one with oats, calendula, and blue malva.

Sunset in Emerald Valley

Here's another favorite evening tea blend, named after the Emerald Valley, where I opened my first herb school, The California School of Herbal Studies, in 1978. Located 16 miles from the Pacific coast, the valley sunsets were colorful affairs.

» 2 parts spearmint leaf
» 1 part hibiscus flower
» 1 part lemon balm leaf
» ¼ part cinnamon chips
» ¼ part gingerroot (fresh grated is best but dried will do)
» A pinch of stevia or honey to sweeten (optional)

To make and use the tea:
Prepare an infusion of the herbs (including the stevia), following the instructions on page 29. Drink a cup or two in the evening after dinner.

This is another of those beautiful garden herbs that early European colonists brought with them to the United States. Also called garden heliotrope, it was both a hardy garden flower planted to remind them of their homeland and a valuable medicine used to reduced pain and stress — and I'm sure there was a lot of that in those early years. Valerian is still considered one of our safest and most powerful herbal nervines, used for all manner of stress, insomnia, and anxiety. It is also excellent for relieving muscle pain. Its name derives from the Latin word *valere*, meaning "to be well" or "to be strong."

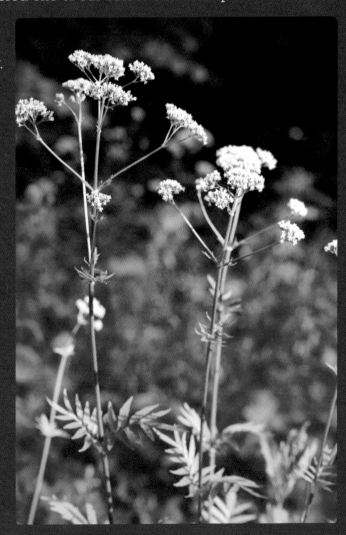

GROWING VALERIAN

Another easy-to-grow perennial, valerian does well in a variety of soil conditions and temperatures. But it prefers partial shade to full sun and moist, rich soil and will thrive if you give it these conditions. It is a rather tall (3 to 5 feet), graceful plant with lacy white flower clusters that bloom through much of the summer. It's hardy to Zone 4, or even Zone 3 if given some winter protection. The seeds are so easy to germinate that even beginner gardeners should have no problem with them. Keep the soil well watered; valerian loves moist soil. Once established, this hardy perennial will self-sow easily and generously. In fact, I'm forever finding valerian popping up everywhere in my garden.

MEDICINAL USES

Valerian is a remedy primarily for stress, tension, insomnia, and nervous system disorders. Studies show that it works by depressing activity in the central nervous system and relaxing the smooth muscles of the uterus, colon, and bronchial passages. Most of the research has focused on the volatile oils found in the roots. Two compounds, valerenic acid and valerenal, have been found to induce sleep and indirectly raise levels of gamma-aminobutyric acid, a neurotransmitter that decreases central nervous–system activity. There's speculation that valerian may work in part because it bonds with receptor sites in the central nervous system. But we don't really know how it works, only that it does. It is effective both as a long-term nerve tonic and as a remedy for acute nerve problems such as headaches and pain.

Valerian also has tonic effects on the heart and is especially recommended in cases of irregular heartbeat and anxiety that affects the heart. It is often combined with hawthorn berry to treat high blood pressure and irregular heartbeat.

Valerian has always been one of my favorite nerve tonics and muscle relaxants. It's the herb I use when I can't fall asleep. And when I wake up in the night and can't get back to sleep, I reach for the valerian tincture, take several dropperfuls, and am generally back to sleep in a few minutes. It's also the herb I use to relieve muscle tension and backache.

Part Used

Root

Key constituents

Isovalerenic acid, valerenic acid, caffeic acid, tannins, sesquiterpenes, glycosides, essential oils, calcium, magnesium, B vitamins

Safety factor

Generally considered safe. However, valerian doesn't agree with everyone and for some people it can be irritating and stimulating, rather than calming and sedating. Avoid taking large doses of valerian for an extended period of time; instead, use modest doses for just 2 to 3 weeks, with a week's break before you begin taking the doses again.

For those people for whom valerian works, it works well. Some people, however, find it irritating and stimulating, rather than relaxing. The root is rich in isovalerenic and valerenic acids, which give it powerful nervine properties. However, some people are unable to process these two acids, and for them, rather than being relaxing, the herb will agitate and overstimulate. You'll know the first time you try it. If you happen to be one of the people for whom valerian is contraindicated, not to worry. The fact that your body can't convert the isovalerenic and valerenic acids doesn't mean there's something wrong with you, only that valerian is not your cup of tea!

Because of the volatile nature of its aromatic oils, valerian root is generally infused rather than decocted. Don't be afraid to take sufficient amounts of this herb; it's nonaddictive and will not make you feel sleepy or groggy. Begin with a low dosage and increase until you feel the relaxing effects. If you take too much valerian, you'll begin to have a rubbery-like feeling in your muscles — like they are *too* relaxed — or a feeling of "heaviness." Cut back the dosage so that you feel relaxed but alert.

Fresh valerian root has an earthy odor that has been likened to that of wet soil or violets. The dried root's odor is more akin to that of dirty socks or a boys' locker room. Depending on the individual, the smell is either relished or deemed offensive. Without a doubt, the taste is better when the root is fresh. Herbalists are in disagreement about whether the fresh or dried herb is more potent medicinally. It's a personal preference, I've found. Regardless, because of the unusual flavor and odor, many people prefer to take valerian in tincture or capsule form, rather than as a tea.

Tension-Free Formula

This formula can be helpful in cases of muscle spasm, heart arrythmia, and anxiety.

» 2 parts valerian root
» 1 part hawthorn berry (or berry, leaf, and flower)
» 1 part lemon balm leaf

To make the formula:
Prepare an infusion of the herbs, following the instructions on page 29, using 1 to 2 ounces of herb per quart of water, and letting the herbs steep for at least 45 minutes or even overnight. Alternatively, tincture the herbs in 80-proof alcohol, following the instructions on page 40.

To use:
For the tea, drink 2 to 3 cups daily. For the tincture, take ½ to 1 teaspoon three times daily, or as often as needed.

Bronchial Relaxer Formula

This formula is helpful for treating deep spastic coughs.

» 1 part licorice root

» 1 part valerian root

» ¼ part cinnamon bark

» ¼ part ginger root

To make the formula:
Prepare an infusion of the herbs, following the instructions on page 29, using 1 to 2 ounces of herb per quart of water, and letting the herbs steep for at least 45 minutes or even overnight. Alternatively, tincture the herbs in 80-proof alcohol, following the instructions on page 40.

To use:
For the tea, drink 2 to 3 cups daily. For the tincture, take ½ to 1 teaspoon three times daily, or as often as needed.

Deep-Sleep Tincture

This is my favorite formula for insomnia.

» 1 part valerian root

» ½ part hops strobile

» ¼ part lavender flower

» 80-proof alcohol

To make the tincture:
Tincture the herbs in the alcohol, following the instructions on 40.

To use:
Take 1 teaspoon an hour before bedtime and another 1 teaspoon just before going to bed. If you do wake up in the night, take 1 to 2 teaspoons, as needed.

Variation

If you are the type of person who can't sleep because you can't stop thinking and your mind spins endlessly, add 1 part skullcap leaf (*Scutellaria lateriflora*) to this formula.

Yarrow / *Achillea millefolium*

Sporting a full head of lovely white flowers above a stem of lacy leaves (its species name, *millefolium*, means "thousand leafed"), yarrow is, as are many medicinal herbs, a common wayside plant found in most temperate climates of the world. Wherever yarrow grows, it has woven its way into the folklore and medicine of the native cultures. It may well be one of the most widely used medicinal plants in the world!

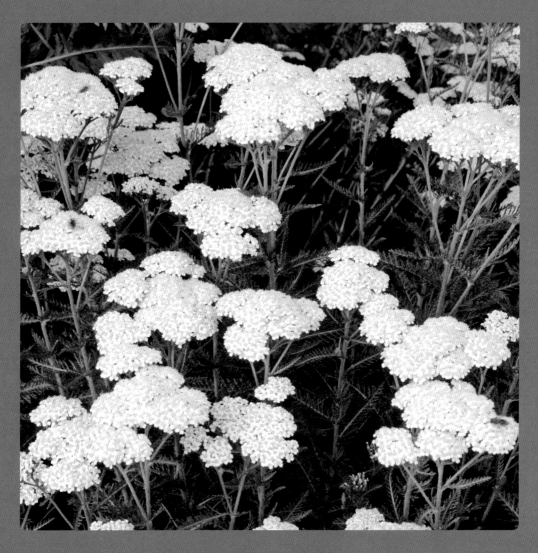

GROWING YARROW

Yarrow grows freely and joyfully in the wild and — whenever it's invited — in the garden. A perennial, it germinates easily from seed and, once established, will self-sow readily. Yarrow will thrive in most types of well-drained soil with a pH of 4 to 7 and prefers full sun, but it happily adapts to a variety of situations: full sun or partial shade, cold or hot weather, wet or dry conditions. For medicinal purposes, look for the wild white yarrow (*Achillea millefolium*) or native pink varieties. The colorful hybrids are bred for aesthetics, rather than medicinal properties. Though it can be harvested throughout the growing season, yarrow has the richest concentration of medicinal oils when it is in flower.

MEDICINAL USES

Yarrow has antiseptic, anti-inflammatory, and astringent properties and is highly regarded for healing wounds, bruises, and sprains. Recently, when herbalist Matthew Wood was visiting my home, one of my students slipped and sprained her ankle quite severely. As her ankle began to swell and turned black and blue, Matthew quietly gathered a handful of fresh yarrow flowers, mixed them with elder flowers, and applied this fresh poultice directly to the swelling. Within a few minutes, literally before our eyes, the swelling subsided and the young woman reported that the pain had diminished substantially.

Like spearmint, yarrow is amphoteric, meaning it moves in the direction it's needed in the body. It is both stimulating and sedative. For example, it is used to

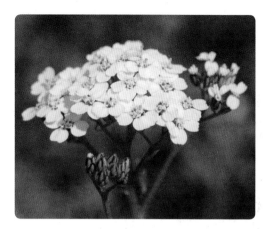

Both the blossoms and the leaves of the yarrow plant are medicinal.

stimulate delayed or absent menstrual cycles and helps ease and relax uterine tension and menstrual cramps. At the same time, it is very effective at reducing heavy bleeding during menstruation. As a uterine relaxant and styptic, it's also a useful aid during childbirth; many midwives today pack their yarrow tincture when attending a birth.

Yarrow is a styptic, meaning that it stops bleeding. It's often mixed with shepherd's purse, another powerful styptic, as first aid to stanch excessive bleeding, whether from a cut, a deep wound, or a simple nosebleed. When my gardener Micki sliced off a small section of her little finger while using a string trimmer one day, blood gushed everywhere. Thankfully, our garden is overflowing with yarrow. Micki took several leaves, mashed them up right there on the spot, and applied a thick poultice to the deep wound. Within minutes the bleeding slowed, and a few minutes later it stopped completely.

Yarrow is rich in volatile oils, specifically chamazulene, camphor, and linalool, which stimulate blood flow to the surface of the skin and aid in elimination via the pores. This helps explain its long-standing reputation as a diaphoretic — an herb that promotes sweating and, thus, can help reduce fevers by "driving out" the heat and naturally cooling the body. I've used yarrow in the bath for this purpose and seen it drive down a high fever within 20 minutes. (The added benefit of the herbal bath is that it helps prevent dehydration, a common problem with a high fever.)

Yarrow also has antispasmodic properties and is used to relieve both menstrual and stomach cramps. It is often combined with ginger for this purpose, whether taken internally or applied topically as a poultice. And finally, taste a leaf of yarrow. It is definitely bitter! Bitter herbs stimulate liver function and aid in digestion by stimulating the secretion of digestive enzymes. No wonder this herb had the nickname "cure-all." It is one of the most versatile and healing plants we can grow in our gardens and is as valuable and useful today as it ever was.

Parts used

Leaf and flower

Key constituents

Linalool, pinene, thujone, camphor, azulene, chamazulene, proazulene, beta-carotene, vitamin C, vitamin E, flavonoids

Safety factors

Generally yarrow is considered safe and nontoxic. But because of its stimulating action on the uterine muscles, it should be avoided during pregnancy, especially the early stages, though it is used at childbirth to facilitate labor and stop excessive bleeding.

Also, yarrow can cause an allergic reaction in some people. Discontinue use if you develop itchy eyes and/or a rash.

Yarrow First-Aid Tincture

Use this tincture to relieve stomach cramps and indigestion, stanch bleeding, and help heal bruising.

To make the tincture:
Tincture fresh yarrow leaf and flower, following the instructions on page 40.

To use:
To use externally, soak a cotton cloth in the tincture and apply directly to the affected area as a poultice. To use internally, take ¼ to ½ teaspoon of the tincture three or four times daily.

Styptic Powder

You'll want to always have a small amount of powdered yarrow available for nosebleeds and those nasty cuts that never seem to stop bleeding.

To make the powder:
Gather fresh yarrow leaves and flowers. Dry them (see instructions on page 19), finely powder the dried herb, and store the powder in a jar or tin.

To use:
Sprinkle a small amount of the styptic powder directly on an open wound to slow the bleeding. To stop a nosebleed, sprinkle a small amount of powder on the inside of the nostril that's bleeding. The powder will usually slow or stop the flow of blood within minutes.

You can also take powdered yarrow internally to help stop the flow of blood. Stir ¼ to ½ teaspoon of the powdered yarrow (or yarrow tincture, if you have it handy) into a small amount of water and drink it down.

Fever-Reducing Tea

This recipe is based on a famous old Gypsy recipe that's been passed around for centuries. It's hard to improve on it, it's so good as it is.

» 1 part elder flower
» 1 part peppermint leaf
» 1 part yarrow flower and leaf

To make the tea:
Prepare a strong infusion of the herbs, following the instructions on page 29.

To use:
Drink ½ cup every 30 minutes to bring on a good sweat. Once you begin to sweat, reduce the amount of tea to ½ cup every hour and continue until the fever subsides.

Yarrow Venous Salve

This salve is especially valuable for distended veins and capillaries, tightening and firming blood vessels, and clearing blood congestion, which makes it useful for treating hemorrhoids, varicose veins, and bruises. Witch hazel bark, should you opt to include it, is an excellent astringent and helps firm and tone tissue.

» 2 parts yarrow leaf and flower (preferably fresh, but dried will do)

» 1 part comfrey leaf

» 1 part witch hazel bark, shredded (optional)

» Olive oil

» Grated beeswax

To make the salve:
Infuse the herbs in oil, following the instructions on page 35. Add the beeswax to the oil, following the instructions on page 38, to turn it into a salve.

To use:
Apply to the affected area several times a day.

Yarrow Liniment for Varicose Veins

With a full complement of astringent, firming, and toning herbs, this simple liniment is very helpful for treating varicose veins and bruises.

» 1 part yarrow flower and leaf

» ½ part raspberry leaf

» ⅛ part cayenne flakes

» Apple cider vinegar (unpasteurized)

To make the liniment:
Place the herbs in a widemouthed jar. Add enough apple cider vinegar to cover them by 2 inches. Cover the jar and let sit in a warm spot for 2 to 3 weeks. Strain and bottle.

To use:
Gently massage the legs up toward the heart, using the liniment and rubbing it in well. Use long, steady, upward strokes only. If the veins are quite extended, soak a cloth in the liniment and apply as a compress directly over the veins. This liniment is helpful for healing bruises as well, but for obvious reasons it is not recommended for hemorrhoids.

Resources

I generally suggest purchasing herbs and herbal products from local sources, as that helps support herbalism and community-based herbalists. However, if you need to search further afield, here are some of my favorite sources for high-quality products.

Herbs

Frontier Natural Products Co-op
844-550-6200
www.frontiercoop.com

**Healing Spirits Herb Farm
& Education Center**
607-566-2701
www.healingspiritsherbfarm.com

**Jean's Greens Herbal Tea Works
& Herbal Essentials**
518-479-0471
www.jeansgreens.com

Mountain Rose Herbs
800-879-3337
www.mountainroseherbs.com

Pacific Botanicals
541-479-7777
www.pacificbotanicals.com

Wild Weeds
707-839-4101
www.wildweeds.com

Zack Woods Herb Farm
802-851-7536
www.zackwoodsherbs.com

Educational Resources

American Herb Association
www.ahaherb.com
Complete listings of schools, programs, seminars, and correspondence courses offered throughout the United States.

American Herbalists Guild
617-520-4372
www.americanherbalist.com
The only national organization for professional, peer-reviewed herbal practitioners; offers a directory of members.

California School of Herbal Studies
707-887-7457
www.cshs.com
One of the oldest herb schools in the United States, founded by Rosemary Gladstar in 1978.

**Sage Mountain Retreat Center
& Botanical Sanctuary**
802-479-9825
https://sagemountain.com
Apprenticeships and classes with Rosemary Gladstar and other well-known herbalists, as well as a home-study course.

United Plant Savers
802-476-6467
www.unitedplantsavers.org
A nonprofit organization dedicated to the conservation and cultivation of endangered North American medicinal plants. Provides conferences, journals, and other educational services to members.

Photography Credits

Interior photography by © Jason Houston: 3, 4, 6, 7, 9, 13, 14, 18, 20, 22–49, 52, 56, 57, 63, 67–69, 72, 75, 80, 81, 85, 93, 101 (row 3, center right; row 4, center left), 104, 105, 110, 114–116, 125, 139, 142, 148, 151, 155, 157, 176, 193, 200, and 207

Additional photography by:

© Elena Schweitzer/iStockphoto.com: 5 (bottom)

© Floortje/iStockphoto.com: 5 (top) and 89

© Bojidar Beremski/iStockphoto.com: 11 (top)

© fotolinchen/iStockphoto.com: 11 (bottom)

© Anna Yu/iStockphoto.com: 15

© Luceluceluce/Dreamstime.com: 16 and 59

© Helena Lovinicic/iStockphoto.com: 51 (middle row right), 64 and 65

© Creative99/iStockphoto.com: 51 (top row left), 53

© AGStockUSA/Alamy: 51 (top row center), 83

© GAP Photos/Graham Strong: 51 (top row right), 94

© GAP Photos/Lynn Keddie: 51 (middle row left), 54, and 90

© Matthew Ragen/iStockphoto.com: 51 (middle row center) and 60

© bokehcambodia/Alamy: 51 (bottom row left) and 78

© GAP Photos/Thomas Alamy: 51 (bottom row center), 86, 101 (row 5 center left), and 144

© Denis Pogostin/iStockphoto.com: 51 (bottom row right) and 70

© Konrad Kaminski/iStockphoto.com: 55

© Aji Jayachandran/Dreamstime.com: 58

© eli_asenova/iStockphoto.com: 61

© Bob Sylvan/iStockphoto.com: 71

© YinYang/iStockphoto.com: 76

© Nigel Cattlin/Alamy: 79 and 204

© ELyrae/iStockphoto.com: 91

© Mark Gillow/iStockphoto.com: 92

© Dinodia Photo Library/Botanica/Getty Images: 95

© Tim Bowden/iStockphoto.com: 97

© Sylwia Kachel/iStockphoto.com: 98

© Galina Ermolaeva/iStockphoto.com: 101 (row 1 left) and 197

© Zorani/iStockphoto.com: 101 (row 1 center left), 129, and 131

© Jolanta Dabrowska/iStockphoto.com: 101 (row 1 center right), 159, and 208

© GAP Photos/Howard Rice: 101 (row 1 right) and 161

© Tim Gainey/Alamy: 101 (row 2 left) and 181

© Rewat Wannasuk/Dreamstime.com: 101 (row 2 center left) and 102

© BasieB/iStockphoto.com: 101 (row 2 center right, row 3 right), 112, and 192

© GAP Photos/Dave Bevan: 101 (row 2 right), 134, and 170

© GAP Photos/Keith Burdett: 101 (row 3 left) and 171 (right)

© Vasiliki Varvaki/iStockphoto.com: 101 (row 3 center left) and 117

© Garden World Images/age fotostock: 101 (row 4 left) and 184

© Gary K. Smith/Alamy: 101 (row 4 center right) and 109

© Bob Gibbons/Alamy: 101 (row 4 right) and 166

© Arco Images GmbH/Alamy: 101 (row 5 left) and 121

© Arterra Picture Library/Alamy: 101 (row 5 center right) and 188

© Uros Petrovic/iStockphoto.com: 101 (row 5 right) and 156

© GAP Photos/Juliette Wade: 101 (row 6 left) and 203

© John Glover/Alamy: 101 (row 6 center left) and 149

© GAP Photos/Pat Tuson: 101 (row 6 center right) and 212

© Sasha Fox Walters/iStockphoto.com: 101 (row 6 right) and 124

© Alberto Pomares/iStockphoto.com: 103

© Andris Tkacenko/iStockphoto.com: 106

© Maximilian Weiner/Alamy: 107

© TOHRU MINOWA/a. collection RF/Getty Images: 108

© Lew Robertson/Botanica/Getty Images: 111

© Maksim Tkacenko/iStockphoto.com: 113

© Andreas Herpens/iStockphoto.com: 118 (top)

© AntiMartina/iStockphoto.com: 118 (bottom), 128

© Elena Eliseeva/iStockphoto.com: 120

© Moehlig Naturfoto/Alamy: 122

© Bildagenturonline/Alamy: 123

© dk/Alamy: 126

© Wally Eberhart/Getty Images: 132 and 133

© Robert Whiteway/iStockphoto.com: 135

© Frans Rombout/iStockphoto.com: 137

© Andersastphoto/Dreamstime.com: 138

© 2009 Steven Foster: 140

© Peter Kindersley/Getty Images: 141 and 191

© Medic Image/Getty Images: 143

© Imbali Images/Alamy: 145

© Anton Ignatenco/iStockphoto.com: 146

© Image Broker/Alamy: 150

© Mashuk/iStockphoto.com: 153

© blickwinkel/Alamy: 162

© Peter Anderson/Getty Images: 165 and 174

© Bon Appetit/Alamy: 169 and 205

© GAP Photos/Marg Cousens: 171 (left)

© Niall Benvie/Alamy: 173

© Magdalena Kucova/iStockphoto.com: 175

© Andrei Nikolaevich Rybachuk/iStockphoto.com: 178

© Westend61 GmbH/Alamy: 180

© Kathryn8/iStockphoto.com: 182

© Lezh/iStockphoto.com: 187

© GAP Photos/Jason Smalley: 189

© John Pavel/iStockphoto.com: 194

© Givaga/iStockphoto.com: 196

© GAP Photos/Fiona Lee: 198

© Kal Stiepel/Getty Images: 199

© Michael Rosenfeld/Getty Images: 202

© dirkr/iStockphoto.com: 209

© Sergey Chushkin/iStockphoto.com: 211

© M & J Bloomfield/Alamy: 213

© nadezzzdo9791/iStockphoto.com: 215

© United Plant Savers: 217

Index

Entries in **bold** indicate a chart.